Anxiety Relief
When You're On-The-Go

Calm Overthinking, Manage Stress, Feel Safe

Christian J. Meadow

Table of Contents

Introduction

You can't always find time to go meditate on a mountain top, but you can practice slow breathing in the shower. – Caroline at LessStressMoreEnergy.com

Is This Guide for You? Christian's Story

I don't know whether my Qigong coach even remembers saying these words, but Caroline's words have helped me overcome many difficult times ever since.

My story might help you decide whether this guide is for you. I am a typical always-on-the-go American. Outwardly I coped, and few people would even have suspected how exhausted I had been before I learned to manage my anxiety. This book is my story but also the story of millions of ordinary hard-working, good people.

Nobody wakes up in the morning and thinks: "I'd like to be anxious and stressed today." On the contrary, most people want to be happy and healthy. Yet, chronic low-level stress, anxiety, and tension are endemic in our lives. Furthermore, they can cause significant health issues, misery, and exhaustion.

I tell you my story not looking for sympathy or recognition but because I believe it can help you to start breathing in the shower and through your busy day.

This guide is for you if you regularly experience any of the following symptoms: irritability, anger, fatigue, nervousness, headaches, sadness, wanting to cry, digestive issues, muscle pain, change in appetite, teeth grinding, and problems with sex.

Anxiety (according to Merriam-Webster) is an abnormal and overwhelming sense of apprehension and fear, often marked by physical signs such as tension, sweating, increased pulse rate, and doubt concerning the reality and nature of the perceived threat.

Ask me; I have been down the anxiety road at such a fast pace that I could barely stop and ask myself: *What is going on?* Fortunately, life stopped me in my tracks. Late one night, I had to ask myself: *How can I change my life? How can I stop feeling anxious and fearful all the time?*

Listening to the unnerving beep-beep of the heart monitor, I decided to sell up and move to Kentucky, where my grandparents once farmed. I saw myself tilling the soil, selling my veggies at a farmers market, and hiking the trails in the foothills of the Appalachian Mountains my grandfather so often talked about.

But life happened. I could not sell up and move. However, on a rainy afternoon, I lost my keys and had to wander around waiting for my neighbor to get home. With rain drizzling down, I had a glimpse through an open door of a group of people standing still, apparently doing nothing. The peace on their faces got me, and I wandered in. The coach waved me welcome, and I followed her voice. Soon I was unaware of being an outsider; something shifted in me.

An unexpected crisis with lost keys brought me to Caroline's Qigong class. I joined to get out of the rain but stepped into breathing-in-the-shower and the art of managing anxiety.

Her remark: "You can't always find time to meditate on a mountain top, but you can practice slow breathing in the shower," amused me. A few days ago, I wanted to move to the Appalachian Mountains for a simpler lifestyle. But I soon realized it was an unattainable dream.

After Qigong class, I went home and walked into the usual chaos: Our two-year-old threw a tantrum. My wife stared with dead eyes at the TV screen. At my wit's end, I tried the breathing thing. When I returned to the lounge, I did not make the usual snide remark to my wife. I took my screaming baby girl and started kissing her neck. She stopped screaming after a while, and we got through the night without further outbursts.

A few days later, before a difficult meeting, I tried the shower-breathing in the men's room and managed not to lose my temper with my cocky colleague. Gradually the breathing-in-the-shower-thing became a habit. I was intrigued and went back to Qigong class.

After that, my life fell apart, but strangely I did not.

Life isn't like the movies—one carefully planned crisis after the other that leads the protagonist along a difficult road into a beautiful future. Unlike movies, life does not follow a neatly organized script that leads to a happy ending. Life often rushes from one unplanned, chaotic moment to the next before it finally crashes in on you.

And even if you can sell up and move to the Rockies, your anxiety will move with you.

In this book, I share how I coped through repeated health scares, divorce, and heartbreak. I want to show you how basic techniques not only saved me but brought me peace while running the rat race. Breathing, acupressure, and Qigong became my go-to coping mechanisms when anxiety engulfed me in darkness and despair.

At the beginning and during the darkest days of my illness and personal upheaval, I switched between them, wondering which one I should embrace. Later, they interweaved into my daily routines, and I discovered I did not have to choose between these techniques. I could selectively do bits and pieces of all three as my circumstances allowed. None of them involves exclusive membership or requires any qualifications.

They gradually became part of my daily routines:

When a bad headache sets in, I would unobtrusively massage the valley in the web between my thumb and index finger.

I breathed slowly in the shower for a few days before the hectic final meeting with my wife and her lawyers.

To keep in practice, I regularly attend Qigong classes.

In this book, I want to help you to:

Use instant techniques in those on-the-go moments when anxiety grips and threatens to overwhelm you.

Practice these techniques at home to teach your body and mind to switch to the instant-technique mode when life gets hard.

Employ the influencing techniques to shift your attitude and sometimes the other person's attitude.

We all have our stories, and although the details differ, I firmly believe that this book's techniques can help you manage your anxiety to have a fulfilling life right where you are and irrespective of your story.

With practice, these basic techniques become second nature. Breathing a loud lion's breath makes me smile. But the smile stays with me for days.

Chapter 1:

My Journey Home

So much time and effort are spent on wanting to change, trying to change, to be somebody different, better, or new. Why not use this time to get comfortable with yourself as you are instead? —Andy Puddicombe

Living Up to Expectations

My first conscious memory was of me, two or three years old, sitting in the church pew with my parents in our Sunday best. I wore a white shirt, navy shorts, a spotted navy blue bow tie, and a matching belt carefully threaded through the loops of my grown-up pants. My mother tried to pat down my unruly curls now and then. My dad frowned when my laced-up boots tupped-tupped into the pew in front of me.

I vaguely remember the other kids kicking a ball after church. My cousin, Geoff, waved and threw the ball invitingly at me. I instinctively knew I could not join in because of the whole bow tie thing. It dawned on me that day that I had to look and play the part my parents chose for my life: well-dressed, well-behaved, not having fun with cousin Geoff and the neighborhood kids.

It became the standard by which I lived my life. I played organized sports after school, not spontaneous ball after church. I studied the subjects my teachers thought were the right ones for a proper career, not art and music like I wanted to. I made friends with the kids from the right part of the rail tracks, not the ones who smoked behind the library.

I went to university, became a lawyer, and married the right girl from a good church-going family. On the surface, I had a good life: a respectable job, a refined wife, and a young family. I lived the life my parents, teachers, and community approved of.

But at night, I woke up sweating with my heart racing. I was constantly tired but had trouble sleeping. I lived a double life: outwardly smiling and confident, inwardly expecting the worst to happen at any moment.

In my rare moments alone, I struggled to breathe. Dizzy and confused, I knew something was drastically wrong, but I did not know what. Was it my strained relationship with my wife? The boredom of being a small-town lawyer? My ailing health?

My Body Spoke Up When I Kept Quiet

Eventually, my body spoke up when I kept quiet. I don't want to bore you with the details: Heart attack number one, divorce, a big mess at work, overlooked for promotion, and heart attack number two. I could no longer continue to live a life where I didn't belong. Yet, I did not know any other life.

Somehow, in the chaos, I realized that when things were hard, I relied on the breathing techniques I had learned in Qigong class. But in my mind, Qigong was still something far removed from real life. Anyhow, how could breathing help when my life is falling apart?

Nonetheless, a Qigong class to kill time and escape the sad drizzling streets was the beginning of an internal shift that I could initially not explain. Even though I could not describe the change in my body and mind, I became a regular at the back of Caroline's class.

The real turnabout came after another life-happens moment. I crashed my car into a lamp post. It was the last thing I needed on that day. It was the first time my children could stay with me for a few consecutive days, something we had all looked forward to very much. I had to postpone their pick-up time, and while waiting for the tow truck, I wandered into the bookshop.

East Met West at the Coffee Shop

He was sitting with a coffee and a stack of books in the coffee nook: My cousin, Geoff, who went somewhere east after university. Ever since, the family spoke in whispers about him, their eyes shifting nervously around to check whether Geoff's parents were within earshot. Some things were never discussed openly in my family. I instinctively knew not to probe Geoff's defiance of our family's tradition of pursuing a professional career and having a stable family life.

But here Geoff was. We hugged and surprisingly started talking as if we still lived on the same street and went to church every Sunday. We laughed and talked about our parents and how far life took us apart. I was a lawyer sitting in the same office as my father did for forty years. He became an English teacher on the other side of the world, a place his father refused to visit.

I saw the book titles and asked about his connection to breathing and healing. Geoff noticed my sallow complexion and asked about my health. He looked me in the eye and said, "You look exhausted. Your medication doesn't seem to work entirely. Would you consider trying Eastern treatments to complement your treatment?"

I was taken aback. I knew nothing about Eastern medicine, let alone that it could complement Western medicine. And for the first time, I admitted to myself and someone else: Yes, I have a heart condition, but my real problem lies much deeper.

I blurted out about the interrupted sleep despite sleeping tablets, the fear that sometimes forced me to pull off the road shivering, and the panic attacks that squeezed the air from my lungs. I am constantly anxious about so many things. I heard myself say, "The only thing that seems to help is my Qigong breathing techniques."

"I'm not surprised," Geoff said. "You are halfway there already. Qigong is much more than breathing techniques. It's the root of life. Without Qi, life is not possible."

But then the tow truck came, and we had to say goodbye. "I'm here most days," Geoff said quietly, and I knew I'd go back.

I fetched my children in a rented vehicle, and we had quality time together for the first time in a long time. However, Geoff's words stayed with me, and I instinctively knew that my inner life had taken a turn for the better.

Looking back at my coffee shop journey with Geoff, I sensed his inner peace but did not understand it. I envied the quiet place within him that I could not quite pinpoint. He was never in a hurry to finish a coffee or to run for a meeting. Little did I know that his calm exterior hid a deep pain.

Only late into our regular chats, Geoff shared that he lost his wife to cancer. He returned to the US because of better educational opportunities for his young son. The immensely talented Billy has Down syndrome.

Geoff's voice broke, and I realized how deep his pain was. He explained how difficult it was to set the borders on Billy's education. He wanted to protect his son from life's challenges but knew Billy had to find his own way.

At a lack for words, I asked, "How do you cope with such worry?"

"I breathe," Geoff said. "I breathe to let go. Every time grief grips me, I breathe deeply, and my lungs help me carry my grief through my entire body, and then they let go. I breathe slowly and deeply and feel my pain intensely, but with a long, thorough exhale, my lungs help the grief exit. I breathe like this whenever grief overwhelms me."

Geoff's answer made me realize I was on to something very real. My regular Qigong class on the other side of town and our frequent coffee chats were more than just interesting breakaways from my routine.

When I looked at Geoff, I wanted to know about the century-old wisdom and science of Eastern philosophy and medicine.

I later learned that in Chinese medicine, the body parts, especially the organs, are much more than the physical object. On top of their respective functions to keep the body healthy and active, they help me release grief from my entire body.

Geoff was exhausted as they had spent most of the previous night in the emergency room at the hospital. He nonetheless seemed calm, telling me how breathing helped him handle his grief.

"Just like I am at the moment, and I suspect you are, the lungs are quite fragile. They are close to the external body and quick to react to sudden drops in temperature, cold wind, also air-conditioners. When I first went to China, I saw a doctor about a nagging chest cold. The man checked my skin. I thought he misunderstood, but my local roommate later explained. The skin and the lungs are connected. A bitingly cold wind dehydrates the skin and may affect the lungs."

"But dehydrated skin might also be a sign of emotional upheaval. It is not something we guys would notice easily. After my wife died, it was as if my tears dehydrated my skin to a sunburnt animal hide."

I did not want to press the issue as I could see Geoff's tiredness, but I read about it later. Eastern healers believe the lungs handle grief as they do with air. They circulate life-giving air through the entire body and then release stale air through the nose. In the same way, they handle grief—they consciously remove it from the body-mind system.

My conversations with Geoff and my weekly Qigong class opened a new world for me. I wanted to know more, experience more and most importantly, enjoy life again. While diligently taking my medication and following the prescribed diet and exercise routine, I steadily learned about the complementary approaches to health and well-being.

Western doctors treat a specific condition; Eastern healers treat the whole person. Both traditions are thousands of years old, and both have a place in health care. People get sick and suffer immense pain and loss because of health problems. Life would be unthinkable without modern medical science.

I am grateful for the medical care I received during my illness. I know it is based on thorough research, clinical trials, diagnostic observation, and carefully evaluated conclusions. Because of a dedicated medical team that treated my damaged heart, I lead a regular and full life.

But Geoff and my Qigong coach alerted me to a complementary healing system, and I wanted to learn more. I put the question to Geoff: "So, how is Traditional Chinese medicine different?"

"After fifteen years of studying first Mandarin and then Chinese traditional medicine, I am still scratching the surface," Geoff said, smiling while sipping his cappuccino.

Once I started reading on the subject, I agreed wholeheartedly. It is impossible to master centuries of wisdom and knowledge in a few years. Chinese medicine is not a single method based on a few basic principles. It includes many therapies, of which I incorporated three into my life: breathing, acupressure points, and Qigong.

Having survived two heart attacks, I was immediately drawn to the Chinese perspective of the heart. Western medicine rates the heart very high in human health. It regulates the rhythm, heart rate, and blood pressure. It pumps oxygen to the lungs and fresh blood to every body part. It removes toxins from the tiniest body cell to the kidneys and carbonated blood to the lungs.

But Westerners also have a different connotation of the hardworking pump in the chest.

Have you ever wondered why Valentine cards and school desks sport a heart with an arrow through it? And the words "heartbroken," "heartsore," and idioms such as "from the bottom of my heart" and "cross your heart and hope to die?" The Western culture is drenched in associated meanings of the all-important heart. We instinctively believe the heart to be the center of feelings and emotions, but this is not typically reflected in Western medicine.

In Eastern tradition, the heart is much more than just a physical organ. It is the center of the human spirit and consciousness and, therefore, the dominant organ. The heart's position in the center of the upper body and its proximity to the diaphragm, lungs, and the fifth vertebrae confirm its importance. The heart is connected to the brain and even the smallest part of the body via the blood vessels. By implication, the heart rules the entire body.

Therefore, on my first visit to a Chinese doctor, he asked about symptoms I would never have associated with my heart health: lethargy, insomnia, constipation, and sore knees. He asked many questions about what basic taste sensation I have in my mouth: salty, sweet, greasy, and only smiled at my skepticism. He looked at my tongue and asked whether I bit my tongue often.

I wondered how my tongue and belly could be related to my heart muscles but did not ask. By that time, I knew my task-orientated, logical mind did not have all the answers—I had a long way to go in understanding the philosophy of traditional Eastern medicine.

But it seemed like the doctor was reading my mind. He placed his fingers on my temples and asked me to breathe slowly in through the nose and out through the mouth. He noticed my reluctance and explained in perfect English, "I want to teach you a simple exercise to ease your tension. This energy channel is called the Triple Heater or Triple Burner in English. In Chinese, we call it Triple Jiao because this is where the energy from all the body parts that regulate your fight-and-flight sense comes together. You can sleep better and improve your anxiety when this energy is calmed."

Anxiety had been part of my being for so long that I was doubtful. However, I have experienced how breathing differently and regularly going to Qigong helped me cope better. I had to try this technique. I had nothing to lose and suspected I had much to gain.

And so I did. If you want to try this, remember that your breath is key here. Practice the finger route in front of a mirror if you want to, but just following your instinct and your breath should be enough.

Calming Anxiety Technique

- ☐ Lying down in a peaceful and dark room, find the spot at your temples right next to the outside of the brows. Making small little circles on the spot helps me anchor my breath.

- ☐ Breathe in deeply through your nose and out through your mouth during the entire routine.

- ☐ Breathe in again and slide your fingers to the ears and around the back of the ears. Retain some light pressure.

- ☐ Breathe out and slide the fingers down the neck to the little valley in the shoulder.

- ☐ Breathe in and press slightly harder into the shoulder.

- ☐ Breathe out and slide the fingers over the heart.

- ☐ Breathe in and out while pressing down firmly.

- ☐ Repeat this as many times as you feel comfortable.

A kind and excellent heart specialist treated my physically broken heart, but the complementary Eastern therapies healed my hidden brokenness. Along the way, my brain learned to react differently to stimuli that previously caused my severe anxiety.

I was puzzled that Geoff, an older cousin and never a close companion during my childhood, was present in many of my life's deciding moments. Geoff challenged me to ignore the bow tie and play ball as a toddler. Geoff casually introduced me to eastern healing when my body was healing, but my soul was hurting. And Geoff alerted me on how to breathe with grief without falling apart.

I found the answer much later and will share it with you in Chapter 6, where I explain how energy in one person may sometimes move the energy in another.

But there is one more episode from the coffee shop that I want to share. It finally won me over. I am not particularly proud of this incident, but the penny finally dropped. Geoff brought Billy to meet me, and we clicked immediately. Something about how Billy looked me trustingly in the eye without judgment stirred me deeply. He asked to see my new car and, excitedly, knocked over his coffee. The manager shouted at Billy, who began to stammer his apologies.

A few drops had spattered across the books in front of Geoff. He immediately got his card out while reassuring Billy and offering to pay.

I felt mindless anger pushing up from my gut and exploding with such intensity that I shocked myself. I could not remember ever being so angry and so verbally abusive. Fortunately, the manager did not push the matter. We finished our coffee, and the manager gave Billy a chocolate muffin on the house. I suppose the manager felt as bad as I did.

On the surface, everything was resolved. But later, when Billy was sound asleep in the back of my car, I apologized to Geoff again.

Embarrassed, I joked, "I don't suppose you have a lung trick to help me with anger?"

Geoff laughed and said, "I am in danger of sounding like the teacher I am, but yes, I have. But I have to ask you something else first. I brought Billy to meet you to see whether he likes you and how you react to him. I have to appoint a legal guardian for Billy, and you came to my mind. The coffee incident decided it for me: You will protect my son when I'm not there."

We had to laugh. An unsavory public outburst ended positively. I loved the idea of a godson and was overjoyed that I was considered good enough to care for Geoff's child. I had indeed come a long way. But the best of all: I had laughed spontaneously for the first time in a long time.

"Okay, Let's not get soppy here. Give me the lung trick for anger," I joked.

"Nope," Geoff replied. "Not the lung, the liver this time."

In Chinese medicine, the liver is not merely responsible for helping with digestion, metabolism, and detoxification. The liver houses the emotions of anger, resentment, frustration, irritability, and bitterness. Geoff shared a little trick with me. Athletes often do this before a competition to release tension from the body. Young kids do it, too, when they need to release emotions.

Release the Five Pumps

- The five pumps refer to the arms, legs, and spine.

- Find somewhere private and do a body shake. Bounce your heels as you shake and pump your arms and hands.

- The sudden shaking increases your breathing rate, and that is fine.

- Shake your body vigorously—even a few seconds may help.

- As you're shaking your body, breathe in through the nose and exhale through your mouth in a long sigh or HAA sound.

- Repeat about five or six times.

- Let the vibrations of shaking reach any points that feel tense, such as your shoulder, jaw, or lower back.

- Keep breathing out through the mouth, letting go of stress and tension.

I grew to love this technique and just hoped nobody at the office ever caught me doing the body shake in the bathroom.

Over the years, I read more about Chinese traditional medicine, but it was the practical experiences and Qigong classes where I learned most.

It took me quite a while to put two and two together. The Chinese doctor and Geoff introduced me to another aspect of traditional Chinese medicine: acupressure.

The body's energy moves along energy pathways called meridians. These pathways are not physically identifiable, but I want to invite you to feel your body energy moving.

Nail Rubbing

- ☐ Hold your hands at chest level.

- ☐ Rub the nails of four fingers, not the thumbnails, vigorously together for 20 seconds. Keep breathing as you do it.

- ☐ Open your hands slowly.

- ☐ You might feel a tingling sensation; your bioenergy is moving.

Your fingertips are at the end of energy pathways (meridians). Stimulating energy flow helps the blood flow as the energy leads the blood. Improving circulation can mean less stress. When muscles are tight, blood and energy flow are impeded. And just for the record: top hairdressers recommend this technique for replenishing the hair follicle and hair growth.

Before even understanding how it works, you feel the energy shift in your body. This shifting of energy is key to the techniques described in this book.

Energy can take form, like our body, or it can be formless, like our thoughts. It's all one energy, manifesting in different ways. Some of it isn't visible to us.

You can't see microwaves, but you still use them daily in your kitchen. You can't see the electromagnetic waves, but you enjoy a late-night program while on a long-distance journey. Science has many mysteries we accept because we experience their benefits: TV, radio, the internet, or a hot meal.

Over the past few years, traditional Chinese medicine changed my life from utter chaos to a meaningful existence. I still have anxiety spells, but now I manage them successfully through the techniques I learned, techniques so simple that I wonder why I have not done them automatically. I am far from completely understanding the Eastern philosophy underlying these techniques. But I am a living example of someone who took the best from both worlds—West and East —to become whole again.

I hope these century-old techniques may also help you find inner peace. I lost so much. I hurt so many people, but above all, I lost years living to others' expectations. I finally came home to myself and experienced a little something of the essence of who I am, before the anxiety of expectations and the experiences of life took effect.

I wish you well on your journey to finding your true, authentic self, and I hope that the techniques in this book will be of some help along the way.

Chapter 2:

Anxiety - How Your Body and Mind Respond

We think we are experiencing reality but what we are really experiencing is our thinking. —Michael Neill

"Fight-or-Flight" Mode

This chapter is for those who'd like to delve into a little bit of the theory. But, if not, feel free to just dive straight into Chapter 3 for more of the practical techniques.

As humans, we're hard-wired to scan for danger continuously. And sometimes, we do need that "fight, flight or freeze" mode switched on to keep us safe. For most of us, the reality is that in modern everyday life, life-threatening physical situations are uncommon. However, in daily life, we experience emotional and psychological threatening situations, which can feel devastating.

Because emotional and psychological issues are hidden, we don't always attend to them as we would have if a lion grabs a child or a rival tribe attacks the village. We suppress the feeling and continue seemingly undisturbed but feeling out of balance with internal tension.

Life can be scary, and many of us have distinct fears, such as public speaking, making a telephone call, attending social gatherings, flying, or meeting in-laws. Many of these fears result from lingering uncertainty and sadness in the psyche. An unexplained fear may be how the subconscious wants to keep you safe. Hidden fears often switch on the body's "fight-or-flight" mode to cope with real or imagined frightening events in our lives.

Sometimes we see any new situation as a threat. Internally, we shoot down anything we can't control or manage: new ideas, strange people, or changes at work. Of course, hesitating about sudden changes is normal, and children are often shy with strangers or new food types.

However, when this tendency continues into adulthood and interferes with everyday life, it can cause immense anxiety. Some of us fear all changes—social, work, moving house, or even a new schedule in public transport. These are red flags signaling potentially debilitating levels of anxiety. Chronic anxiety, fear, tension, and stress may result in the body remaining too much in "fight-or-flight" mode.

Our bodies react instinctively and, often, unknown to us on a conscious level. You might find yourself stamping on the car brake when you are a passenger, your shoulders creeping up to your ears with tension, your jaw clamped shut, and your breathing rapid.

Our bodies are amazing. If we pay attention to the sensations in our body, we notice if our shoulders are uncomfortable. We also notice if our heart is beating fast, our breath is short and shallow, or if we feel light or fatigued. It is the body telling us we're tense.

Maybe if you're feeling foggy, you can take a break, get some fresh air and drink water to clear your head. But, if you are unaware of what your body is telling you, it must shout louder. So, you might get pain, like a headache.

Anxiety in the Body

In tense situations, the body's nervous system reacts to prepare for "fight-flight" mode. But what is "fight-or-flight?" Is it a mental or a physical reaction?

The stress response begins with our thoughts, eyes, or ears noticing danger. They send a message to the brain. Several parts of the brain and the body are involved, and they kick off a series of physical processes. The following happens in a flash:

- ☐ The amygdala receives the visual or sound message and signals the hypothalamus about the impending danger. The hypothalamus is the brain's emotional control room. It communicates with the body through the nervous system.

- ☐ The sympathetic nerves carry the danger signal to the adrenal glands.

- ☐ The adrenal glands prepare the body for action by releasing the stress hormones adrenaline and cortisol.

- ☐ Adrenaline triggers the blood vessels to divert blood to the primary muscles.

- ☐ The breath rate increases, supplying more oxygen via the lungs to the brain and the body.

- ☐ The heart beats faster, distributing fresh blood with oxygen to the muscles to prepare them to fight off the perceived danger.

Usually, when the danger is averted, the body and brain return to their normal state. The person calms down, and life continues at a normal pace.

I suspect I was in a state of "fight-or-flight" for most of my life simply because I was never *at home* in my life. I was constantly trying to please others, to be the perfect son, student, employee, and husband. I was never comfortable in any of these roles. I just never fit the mold.

I suspect many of you might have had similar experiences. Does this scenario sound familiar?

- ☐ Do you tend to internally ask "what if" questions or make sweeping negative statements about your abilities to handle something?

☐ Do you regularly experience physical symptoms such as fatigue, heart palpitations, muscle aches, trembling, dry mouth, sweating, and shortness of breath?

☐ Are you continuously milling around the same thoughts and worries in your mind, fighting the same imaginary fight over and over?

Anxiety in the Brain

Cortisol can affect the brain's function in many ways when the body is under long-term stress. It involves the connectivity between neurons which leads to a loss of sociability and even self-isolation. Prolonged stress may even shrink the prefrontal cortex, which influences memory and learning.

Stress leads to the amygdala—the brain's antenna scanning for impending danger—becoming bigger. It becomes more receptive to danger signals, thus increasing emotional triggers, a vicious cycle leading to anxiety.

Uncontrolled stress hormones and their cumulative reaction in the body may also contribute to heart disease, high blood pressure, and diabetes.

Fortunately, the brain has an exceptional ability that medical doctors call neuroplasticity—the way neural pathways in the brain re-form and rejuvenate themselves. Damaged and tired neurons find new routes to connect and activate brain function. I guess this has happened physically in my brain since I started my journey to minimize anxiety. I am physically and mentally healthier than in previous years.

I pride myself on adapting a few simple techniques to use at the office. The techniques in this book are all simple. The tricky bit is just breaking the mold and doing them. Always stop if your body tells you, though.

A quick trick is to do a shoulder roll while in a zoom meeting. The shoulder roll relieves the physical tension in the shoulder and the neck. The movement increases blood flow to the area, which is vital if you sit in front of a computer for long stretches. If you have shoulder issues, you might need to adapt the technique, go slower, and do much smaller circles. It's about letting the energy flow smoothly. Remember, everybody is different—find what works for you.

Shoulder Roll

☐ Check that your computer camera is switched off.

☐ Stand up with the spine aligned while still listening to the online speaker.

☐ Pull the shoulders to the ears and slowly roll them backward, down, and forward in slow circles.

☐ Keep the forearms at a 90°angle.

☐ Let the palms circle as well, up and down. The hands are powerful vessels for receiving and retaining energy.

In this book, I aim to introduce you to more simple and quick techniques to help you manage anxiety and its impact on your body. Ultimately, the idea is to create a shift that enables you to feel much lighter and happier.

Anxiety in the Mind

How often do you think:

☐ What if she turns me down?

☐ What if I fail?

☐ What if it goes wrong?

☐ What if they don't like me?

Closely related to "what if" questions are negative statements such as:

☐ I'll never succeed.

☐ I am not good enough for this.

☐ I am too old/young/stupid/unsophisticated.

The mind creates negative scenarios, a series of horror movies where you are constantly the loser. These mind movies usually feature imaginary scenarios of things going wrong. Also, the mind seems to dwell on previous insults or wrongs to the extent that negativity may take over and can become a person's default state of mind.

It is not surprising that the mind's default mode is predominantly negative. After all, it is the mind's job to scan for danger. Neuroscientific evidence proves that human brain cells react stronger to negative than to positive stimuli. This tendency comes from the times when humans had to survive many environmental and physical dangers.

In modern times, the human brain still registers bad experiences more intensely than good ones; thus, the tendency to first notice the negative. Psychologists call it negativity bias and warn that, when uncontrolled, it can have adverse effects on behavior, decisions, and relationships.

For years, I did not want to join in the neighborhood's annual street party because someone remarked lawyers were taking everybody for a ride. It was a silly joke that stuck with me for far too long. I made a big issue out of nothing and deprived myself and my family of a pleasant group of people.

I thought it was only me being oversensitive. To my surprise, I discovered it often happens in relationships. Most humans are negatively biased and tend to expect the worst from other people. We may be on the defensive going into a meeting or decide beforehand that our idea will be shot down. This negativity may cause unnecessary confrontation and lead to bad decisions.

When I recede into negativity, I try slowing my breathing and breathing through my nose, to restore my mental balance. Breath is directly linked to the brain's activities, and most people subconsciously use one nostril more than the other in normal breathing. Alternate nostril breathing forces one to use both nostrils equally and breathe deeper. Oxygen moves more fluently to the brain and restores balance and focus. It is also a good exercise for blocked sinuses.

Alternate Nostril Breathing

In this exercise, you switch between nostrils while pressing lightly on the acupressure point right in the center of your head between the eyes. It might feel odd the first time, but give it a go. You can also do this lying down and struggling to sleep.

- [ ] Cover the left nostril with your pinky finger and inhale right.

- [ ] Cover the right nostril with your thumb and exhale left.

- [ ] Inhale left.

- [ ] Switch again and exhale right.

- [ ] Inhale right, and so on.

If your nostril is blocked, breathe very lightly through it and breathe normally in between whenever you need to. You can also use an alternative breath technique, like the ones in the next Chapter. Repeat for about two minutes, keeping the breath slow and relaxed. Once you are into the slow rhythm, feel the calm settling in your mind—more about this in Chapter 3.

Overthinking

We overthink when we turn around the same thoughts in our minds without making progress or solving anything.

Overthinking usually involves several "what if" questions accompanied by negative emotions: self-doubt, anger, jealousy, worry, or grief. Milling past injustices or future concerns around the mind can create stress. If you tend to overthink, as most of us do, you might recognize the overriding sensation of being stuck in the mud—not moving forward.

We have a relationship with our past and the future. Because we are engineered to scan for danger continuously, we move our attention to what we don't like. But if we dig through the mud, we can find treasures and hold on to them instead of keeping the mud and throwing away the nuggets of gold.

It is the same when we think about the past or worry about the future. Instead, we can focus on what we will be grateful for. When we steer a car and turn the steering wheel in a direction, the car automatically follows. Similarly, we can guide our thoughts and energy with attention.

It is often not outside factors that keep us stuck in mind mud but our tendency to analyze something endlessly. There is even a term for it: analysis paralysis.

Remember, you can't control the world, but you can start with your thoughts. Thoughts will always pop up, but the following technique may help you calm the monkey chatter.

Balanced Numbers

A quick tip to anchor the mind is using your senses. I believe these seemingly meaningless actions may help get you out of the mud of negative thinking, calmer, and onto more productive thought processes.

- ☐ Stand still for a moment and see five things. Name and count them deliberately.

Abinger Village Stores
01483 285661

Andrew

283 3 42

☐ Still standing, close your eyes, and hear five things. Once again, name and count them.

☐ Now it is time to use an often neglected sense: Touch.

☐ Feel five things while you describe the texture of touch, such as soft, cold, velvety, smooth, or rough. Try to find your description of the different textures.

The previous quick exercise hopefully brought you a moment of mental quietness. The following technique helps guide our attention and energy.

Technique to Guide Attention and Energy

☐ Try to calm your mind by breathing deeply. Anchoring yourself into breathing may help to reframe your thoughts.

☐ Notice your surroundings: The chair in which you sit, the bed on which you lie, the way the sun catches your feet, or the touch of the breeze on your face. No judgment, no wishing you were somewhere else, just notice.

☐ Get comfortable in your body. Relax your shoulders by lifting them to your ears and lowering them. Relax the jaw and wipe the frown from between your eyes.

☐ Breathe slowly in and out through the nose.

☐ You are now fully present in the moment. Go back to all the gems in your past—all the things you are grateful for. Don't rush it; let your attention go to all the pleasant life experiences.

☐ Come back to the present. Notice the chair again, feel the texture of the upholstery, and the sounds outside the window.

☐ Feel your breath—inhale deeply, exhale slowly.

- You are now ready to direct your attention to the future. Where do you want to go?

- Your beautiful mind can move through space and time. You can guide your energy with your mind.

- Create a mind movie of all the things you hope for. Your mind is like a sculptor; you can be the artist of your own life.

- Now, get a bit more real: See it, feel it, hear it. Let your heart expand and open it. We feel joy when we attract positive energy to us.

- Bring this energy back to the present moment. Feel the chair and the floor under your feet. Have a sense of gratitude and excitement for what is to come, the wonderful energy flowing through your body.

- Center all this energy by holding your hands over your lower abdomen.

- Breathe slowly and deeply, settling this happiness and gratitude in your being.

What Is Your Default?

Strangely, nobody needs to teach us to worry. But we have to consciously train ourselves not to worry. Switching from worry mode to relax mode does not come easily.

When you feel emotionally exhausted, reading about and trying out the breathing techniques in the next chapter might be a good idea to help you relax. It might be necessary to try different breathing patterns to find one that works for you.

Basic Breathing to Feel Calm

I often do this basic breathing technique at my desk without anyone noticing.

- ☐ Inhale slowly and deeply.

- ☐ Exhale while you count to five.

- ☐ Repeat this pattern but try to lengthen your exhale until you reach maybe ten counts or whatever feels comfortable. Don't overstretch yourself.

If you feel calmer, you're likely to be more objective. It is a good time to look for "what if" thoughts and ungrounded sweeping statements. Try switching your mind to observer mode and identify those "what ifs" in your mind.

Don't worry or blame yourself for these negative thoughts. It is normal, and most people experience them. However, if your tendency toward negativity means you spend a lot of time in stress mode, regular slow breathing may help you shift the negativity.

When the body's sympathetic nervous system is switched on, all your energy races to the muscles, ready for you to take flight. When you feel you don't have control as a passenger in the car, your body "reads" the message that it's in danger. Your body reacts as if you are racing over a steep cliff on a mountain pass.

If your body is constantly in this danger-ready mode, it has no time to keep your body cells healthy, digest your food properly, or prepare your mind to switch off for proper sleep and rest. In this state, the body does not regenerate cells, do repairs, or deal with diseases. Instead, its priority is fighting or fleeing, which is perfectly fine when standing on a cliff edge or walking down a dark alley. However, your body needs to function at a normal rate during your regular everyday routines.

When fight-or-flight mode is your default, your body is holding chronic low-grade tension. This low-grade tension depletes your energy and spirit. You won't have any reserves to do the things that you enjoy. Robbed of your vitality, you can feel low and sometimes depressed. You may be irritable and snappy and say things that don't really resonate with your true self.

Unwell, exhausted, or in pain, we don't present the best version of ourselves to the world.

In order to relax, the body has to move from fight-or-flight mode (sympathetic nervous system) to "rest and rejuvenate" (parasympathetic nervous system). The sympathetic nervous system kicks in when danger is perceived. The parasympathetic network of nerves relaxes the muscles so the body can rest and heal. The body has to be relaxed for many life-sustaining functions to work properly.

Many processes in the body benefit from a relaxed state in which the body can concentrate on its normal functions. Eyesight improves, salvia in the mouth forms to assist digestion, lung function lessens, the heart beats slower, and natural digestion, urination, and defecation improve.

Feeling grounded, calm, happy, joyful, blissful, grateful, and loved should be our normal default. Deep down, all of us want that. Some seek it consciously, and sometimes we seek it in the wrong places.

Although we can't always be happy, we can at least allow ourselves to flow along with the slipstream of life's ups and downs. A newborn baby is not tense and anxious; we're not born that way. So, releasing stress and anxiety is a step in the direction to re-find that ideal default, your true authentic energy, without conditioning, without the heavy energy of other people, the news, the messy environment, thoughts of the past, and worries about the future.

Email Apnea

Have you heard of email apnea? Sleep apnea is a well-known condition where one temporarily ceases breathing. But scientists have identified another form of unconsciously holding the breath or breathing shallowly and rapidly: email apnea.

Neuroscientists report that when someone focuses intently on something, their brain temporarily switches off some other necessary functions to focus more intensely on the matter. Unfortunately, digital technology can be intellectually and mentally overwhelming. Researchers found that many people hold their breath or go into shallow chest breathing when digitally overloaded.

On the surface, it does not seem serious, as the person resumes breathing at some stage. However, holding the breath regularly or shallow chest breathing alerts the brain of impending danger and causes stress. It can even become a chronic condition that contributes to anxiety.

Take a mental break with this finger-breathing exercise. It is super simple, and you can do it anywhere. It's brilliant to keep the kids (and yourself) calm during a long journey.

The key here is the rhythm between breath and finger movement. Trace up and down each finger, inhaling while going up and exhaling while coming down. But you are not going to rush: There is a short pause at the top of each finger and in the web between the fingers.

Five-Finger Breathing

- Hold one hand in front of you like a starfish.

- Use your index finger on the other hand.

- Start at the thumb and inhale while you move your finger up the outside of the thumb.

- Pause at the top.

- Move your finger down the inside of your thumb while you exhale.

- Pause at the bottom between the two fingers.

- Inhale while your finger moves up the next finger.

- Pause at the top.

- Exhale while you move your finger down.

- Pause in the web.

- Finish one hand and repeat, or switch hands.

- Give your hands a slight shake and feel the calmness settle in your mind.

What happens is that you anchor your mind in your breath. The slower breathing rate signals the brain that the body is safe, and both body and mind relax.

The teasers in this chapter are quick to do and might help you in agitated moments in your daily life, leaving you more relaxed and energized. You will find more techniques to lessen anxiety and stress in the following chapters, as well as how to energize yourself, clear your mind, and balance your emotions.

I provide you with ways to integrate these techniques into your daily life. People doing only ten minutes a day of Qigong, acupressure, or breathing techniques often find a noticeable shift in their anxiety levels even within a few days. I challenge you to do these simple techniques on the bus, at your desk, and at home. Integrate them into your daily life, and experience how your energy shifts and your emotions lift.

As my Qigong coach said during my first class, *you can't always sit on a mountain top and meditate*. Life is demanding. Responsibilities and daily chores leave little time for meditation or quiet moments. In the following few chapters, you'll find lots of simple techniques. You can pick the ones that you like and use them even when you are busy and on the go.

Chapter 3:

Breath Changes Everything

Breath is the Bridge Which Connects Life to Consciousness, Which Unites Your Body to Your Thoughts. Whenever Your Mind Becomes Scattered, Use Your Breath as the Means to Take Hold of Your Mind Again. –Thich Nhat Hanh

The Breath Connects Body and Mind

Just check in with your breathing for a second or two. Don't judge it as good or bad. Whatever you feel is okay. How is your breath at the moment? Is it fast and shallow? Is it slow and deep? Does it feel like it's up in your chest? Is it down in your belly?

Congratulations! You've just achieved the first step toward lessening your anxiety. Yes, the first step is just noticing your breathing. Why? Because this is what just happened: Firstly, for a few seconds, your mind stopped thinking, imagining, and endlessly looping "what ifs." Instead, your mind went into your body to pay attention to your breathing. When your mind notices what's happening now, your mind is in the present moment. When it's in the present moment, it's not reliving the past or worrying about the future.

Secondly, you might have noticed that when you attached your mind to your breathing, your breathing naturally started to change and slow a little. Try it again. Just notice your breathing; put your mind there. When your breathing slows, your nervous system "reads" this as a message that you're okay and that it's safe to relax. Your body can start doing repairs to regenerate your cells. So, just by letting your attention rest on your breathing, you're doing something healthy for your body.

Noticing your breath is a powerful tool we can build on.

Right now, you may find that part of your mind is saying something like this: "Seriously? You're not telling me that something so simple changes my physiology. That's ridiculous. It's too simple. And, anyway, that was just a few seconds."

It sounds familiar, right? Don't worry. As I explained in the previous chapter, we are hard-wired for negativity. It's our default, partly because our subconscious is trying to do an excellent job of keeping us safe. If this happens, just go back to noticing the breath. Anchor yourself in your breath.

It might be a good time for a bit of scientific evidence. Many researchers agree that breath influences several brain regions directly linked to emotions. When you change your breathing rate and patterns, these brain networks are activated and can change your mood, attention, and body awareness.

From the previous chapter, we know increased breathing activates the amygdala and triggers emotions such as irritability, fear, anger, and even anxiety. However, this is not the only effect fast breathing has on the brain and emotions. Researchers also report that we are more attuned to fear if we breathe fast. Yes, rapid and shallow breathing alerts us to fearful situations.

Physical Benefits of Slow Breathing

Slow breathing expands the lungs and increases oxygen flow to the cells in your body. Cells regenerate when they receive fresh oxygen, which gives us more energy. Slow breathing strengthens the lungs and heart; increased blood flow massages the organs and strengthens the muscles. It supports the entire cardiovascular system.

With slow breathing, the parasympathetic nervous system kicks in, and the body calms down. The blood vessels dilate, and blood pressure decreases. Fresh blood washes out toxins, and the immune system becomes stronger.

Slow breathing also improves digestion and helps with weight control. Notice when you breathe slowly and deeply: Your spine lengthens, and your posture improves.

When we are in pain, the muscles tense up, holding on to pain. Slow breathing relaxes the muscles, and the brain releases endorphins, the feel-good hormones.

Emotional Benefits of Slow Breathing

No wonder slow breathing is our go-to technique in times of tension or to combat anxiety. Slow and regulated breathing activates the insula. The insula deep inside the brain regulates, among other things, body awareness. Body awareness (kinesthesia) is the connectedness between your mind and body. When I asked you to check in with your breath, you took the first step in body awareness, but let's try together to sharpen our body awareness.

Body Awareness

☐ Notice how you breathe; don't try to change it. It is okay as it is.

☐ Notice how you feel; don't worry if you feel anxious or even foolish. Your feelings are valid in your present situation. Just go with it.

☐ Sense how the blood flows through your veins, spreading into every part of your body.

☐ See your posture in your mind's eye: Is your back aligned or curved? Are your hands clenched or open? Is your jaw tight or comfortable? What happens to it when you take a slow breath?

☐ Now use your breath to connect and harmonize the body and mind. See how your different body parts, mind, and breath are linked.

I now introduce you to several breathing techniques as tools to manage your emotions and, specifically, to lessen anxiety. Let's continue with abdomen breathing, as this is easy to do anywhere and very effective if you need to calm down.

Abdomen (Belly) Breathing

- ☐ Check your breathing again.

- ☐ Place your hands over your lower abdomen to feel what's happening.

- ☐ When you inhale, let the belly expand like a balloon filling with air.

- ☐ When you exhale, let the belly relax back toward the spine.

- ☐ Do this in a nice relaxed way, not forced. A comfortable, relaxed pace, just a small belly rising and falling, is absolutely fine.

- ☐ It might take a few practice-goes. If you're finding it tricky at first, don't worry; you're doing very well breathing all day long. This is just adjusting it to make it optimal.

- ☐ You can try lying on your back to do it and feel the belly rise as you inhale and relax as you exhale. You can do it anywhere: The bed or the bath is a good place to try it, too. Or when you're outside, opening a window, opening the laptop, walking the dog, as you put down the phone, or as you're feeding the fish.

- ☐ Give yourself time to get used to it, and if you feel it's not working, just shrug, smile and try it again later in the day.

- ☐ A few slowish breaths into the belly whenever you can during the day helps gently retrain the body-mind system.

Congratulations! You've just achieved the next step toward less anxiety.

Why? Because this is what just happened: Like before, your mind stopped whirling for a few seconds while focusing on what's happening. Then you deliberately, consciously, started to slow your breathing just a little. You exercise the diaphragm muscle, which goes up and down in a stretchy-er way when you breathe more into the belly. So, you're starting to train yourself in a new way of breathing, which is healthier and calmer.

When we breathe briefly into our chest, we feel panicky because that's what we do when we're in flight or fight mode. When you consciously shifted your breathing to your belly and slipped into a more relaxed pace, your nervous system got the "everything's okay" message, and you started to feel a little bit lighter.

Nose or Mouth?

If you've come across breathing techniques before, you'll know that some experts advocate breathing through the nose. Others encourage exhaling through the mouth. So, what's the best way to go? Nose or mouth?

Well, it depends.

During a typical day, we should always breathe through the nose. The nose cavities are designed to help you breathe effectively. There are many benefits to nostril breathing and several essential bodily functions. The most obvious one is that the nostrils are excellent filters. They deal with most pathogens and dirt before it gets any further.

The cavities warm the breath you inhale, and when the air reaches the body, it is closer to your body's temperature. Also, your nose releases nitric oxide, which helps widen blood vessels. So, in daily life, breathe in and out through your nose all day and all night long, too.

If you find it difficult to breathe when practicing, try taking very gentle, slow, fine breaths of air in and out through the nostrils. Of course, it is difficult to breathe through your nose when you have a cold, a persistent allergy, or enlarged adenoids.

Temporary mouth breathing is sometimes necessary to get the air to your lungs. You might find your mouth gets dry, and your voice becomes hoarse. It's usually also tiring and might even contribute to bad breath.

However, we sometimes use deliberate, conscious exhaling through the mouth for short sequences to release tension and stale or "stagnant" energy to let go and cleanse. There is some excellent research on this topic, revealing the connection between mouth breathing and sleep apnea, other sleep issues, and sinus infection. James Nestor's great book *Breath* (2020) might be helpful. On the whole, nostril breathing is the way to go.

You're doing great with some slow belly breathing through the nose at intervals during the day. However, sometimes we deliberately want to deviate from nostril breathing and consciously practice mouth breathing for specific reasons, like when we want to release unwanted emotions. We pick this up again in Chapter 5.

Now, let's introduce a little movement along with the breathing, with some relaxing Qigong Flows. Synchronizing breath and movement helps to reset the nervous system.

Opening the Flow

- ☐ Stand firmly grounded, knees relaxed, your spine aligned, and comfortable.

- ☐ Inhale through your nose as you float your arms up in front of you with your palms facing down and wrists relaxed.

- ☐ Exhale, relax the shoulders, drop the elbows, and let the arms float down.

- ☐ Repeat this for two to three minutes.

When we breathe in and out through the nose, we have the intention of circulating life force energy within the body. The following practice, Buddha Holds Up the Earth, helps us expand the chest, lungs, intercostal muscles, and diaphragm and stretch the lung energy pathway.

Buddha Holds Up the Earth

- ☐ Stand with your feet shoulder-width apart, with your spine aligned but comfortable. Beware of locking the knees.

- ☐ Have your palms facing up, just a touch under your navel.

- ☐ Inhale slowly through your nose and feel your spine lengthening as you float your hands, palms up, up the front of the body

- ☐ Turn the palms upward over your head so your thumbs look up to the sky.

- ☐ Pause your breath, and pull your elbows back a little bit, opening the chest.

- ☐ Slowly exhale through the nose as you turn your palms in and float them down the body's front. Repeat for two to three minutes.

These two Qigong and breathwork combined exercises are great to do at home. But, how can we use breathing when life "happens" and we start to feel anxious or stressed? This book's purpose is to use different techniques to counteract anxiety and stress. The first step is to keep practicing slow belly breathing through the nose. We need the practice because it helps us to effortlessly slip into this way of breathing when needed.

It also helps to begin and end your day with a few slow breaths. So, when the alarm goes off in the morning, you can press snooze and do box breathing for a few minutes. It calms your mind, decreases stress, and increases your ability to concentrate. It sets you up for the day.

Box Breathing

- ☐ Lie on your bed (or sit in a chair). If you are sitting, place your feet on the floor, relax your belly and raise the crown of your head toward the sky.

- ☐ Breathe normally for a minute while you shift your awareness to the rise and fall of your belly.

- ☐ Breathe in, counting to four in your mind.

- ☐ Hold your breath for four in your mind.

- ☐ Slowly breathe out while counting to four.

- ☐ Pause your breath for about four.

- ☐ Repeat the last four steps of box breathing for a few minutes or as time allows.

When the alarm goes off again, you're good to go, having set up a calm breathing pattern to start your day. You can repeat this breathing technique at the end of the day too.

My personal bedtime favorite is similar to box breathing. But instead of counting, I imagine waves gently coming in toward the shore, guiding the rhythm of my breathing. So, as I inhale, I hear and see the sea in my mind. There's a pause at the top of the inhale, like the lull before the wave rolls out. But I don't count. Instead, I wait until the breath wants to happen by itself, then I melt into the exhale. There's another lull at the bottom of the exhale, like the sea before the wave comes into shore. And, again, I wait for the inhale to start by itself and just relax right into it.

Let's take this step by step, but don't force it. Go with the flow and let your imagination see it, hear it, feel it, and maybe even smell the salt sea air, to lead you to calmness.

Wave Breathing for Sleeping

- ☐ Lie comfortably.

- ☐ Raise and lower your right shoulder, then the left. Then raise your head and lower it. Feel your spine comfortably aligned.

- ☐ Settle snugly into your bed and relax your body.

- ☐ Bring your right hand to your upper chest and span your thumb and index finger from collarbone to collarbone.

- ☐ Notice your breath but do not worry if it is tense or fast. Just notice how your breath eventually settles down.

- ☐ Close your eyes, or gently gaze ahead but do not focus on anything.

- ☐ Turn your mind to a picture, the sounds, or the feelings of a beach where the waves roll in and out without drama.

- ☐ See, or hear the wave reaching the beach, spreading softly sideways and receding to the ocean.

- ☐ Experience this mind video; try to match your breath to the waves rolling in and out. But, don't try too hard.

- ☐ Allow the waves to roll in and out; your breath automatically catches the rhythm sooner or later. Just let it find its own flow.

- ☐ Notice the slight lull when the wave breaks and follow with the breath.

- ☐ Exhale as the wave rolls back, and notice the pause as the next wave approaches. Let your breath follow this lull.

So, this is where the step-by-step approach stops. It is different for everybody because that twilight zone between awake and sleeping is fragile. Only you can go there. I won't try to guide your wave technique any further. Make it your own and sleep well, knowing that wave after wave will come and go, sometimes with force, sometimes in peace, but always in a never-ending cycle. You can change your mind-movie to suit you.

Congratulations! You've just achieved the next step toward less anxiety.

Why? Because this is what just happened: You've started to train yourself to breathe in a relaxed way using box and wave breathing, and you're regularly practicing morning, evening, and whenever you think of it during the day.

Like most skills and techniques, it does take practice, though. But we've built the practice right into your life, so it doesn't add to your time-consuming to-do list. Initially, you might need reminders, such as post-its around the house and by the bed. Who'd have thought we'd need a post-it to tell us to breathe?

But, after a while, it'll become more of an integrated and automatic part of your daily routine, which is what we want to happen. We'll get to the bit about using this technique in stressful situations next. But first, give it some time, practice. Breathe slowly a couple of times whenever you have a moment: morning, evening, and in-between. If you give it time, you'll start to notice a subtle shift inside you and just a little bit less inclination toward stress.

One of the reasons we're a stressed society is due to our hastiness. We rush around a lot and expect things to be instantaneous. By slowing our breathing, we start to slow our minds, and our stress goes down a notch. When you're able to notice this and put your conscious attention on your breathing, you might perceive a subtle shift; with practice, you'll find it much easier to "switch" at will when we introduce techniques to use in actual stress situations.

But, don't worry if you're not sure, it's totally normal. Just follow along, keep practicing, and you'll get there. Patience with ourselves is the opposite side of the coin to hastiness. Therefore, unsurprisingly, we get impatient for quick results, which can also stress us out. If you start to feel impatient or frustrated, slow your breath and let your mind follow it. Just keep going back to the breath. In the meantime, here's the next step.

Notice Stillness

When you're box or wave breathing, there's a pause or lull at the top of the inhale, followed by another pause at the bottom of the exhale. Now, this time when your breath is still, notice that your mind is still. To start with, just observe this brief stillness in your mind. Take your time; it can take some practice to tune in because we're not used to it. Once you've noticed that the mind is still, just wriggle your way into that stillness so that you can bask in it for a few brief moments before the conscious mind kicks in and starts to question it.

You'll love the experience of this amazing stillness when you start to notice it. It's a moment of serene calm and quiet, a moment of bliss. Don't worry if it doesn't appear to be working. Give it time. Noticing sometimes lies under our consciousness for a while. In the meantime, relax into the brief stillness of the breath filling the belly each time; it has the same calming effect on your physiology.

Congratulations! You've just achieved the next step toward less anxiety.

Why? Because this is what just happened: By noticing what's happening in your body and mind, you're anchoring your mind in the present moment. It may only be brief before the mind's chatter kicks in again, but that doesn't matter. Most of the time, our thoughts about the past or the future trigger our anxiety. Our minds are very busy making elaborate movies that feature things that may never happen, "what ifs," or we focus on the negative experiences of the past and replay them over and over.

But, when we anchor our mind in the present moment, we give it a rest from imagining the future and replaying our perceptions of the past. In the present moment, sitting there in your chair, reading this book, you're probably not in any life-threatening situation. In the present moment, your heart is beating, and your lungs are breathing; you're okay, safe. So, when you noticed your breathing and the stillness between your breaths, your mind was on what was happening there and then. Your mind was in the present moment. Our physical body is only ever in the present moment. It's only our thoughts that travel to the past and the future.

They are thoughts only. They're not embodied. The problem is that the mind doesn't perceive any difference between what we imagine, i.e., our thoughts, and what is really happening in the present moment. So, when we contemplate all the things that we think will go wrong, we paint ourselves a scary, worrying or stressful scene. Our nervous system switches into sympathetic mode. Our body creates fight-or-flight, anxiety, and stress responses because it perceives a real threat from our mind-movie.

Now that you're slowing your breathing and noticing your breath and body regularly during the day, you can start to use the sensation of calm to switch out of anxiety and stress. You've noticed it, so you know what it feels like.

Try this: Think about an apple. What happens? You can see an apple in your mind, right? But it's not actually there. If I cut open your head, I wouldn't find the apple! It's a thought; that apple is just a thought. Now switch that thought from an apple to an elephant.

Changing Thoughts

Congratulations! You've just achieved the next step toward less anxiety.

Why? Because this is what just happened: You changed your thoughts. You were thinking of an apple and changed it to an elephant at will.

Maybe you're feeling anxious about that presentation you have to do tomorrow. You think you won't be able to sleep because of it and that you "know" that the guy from Marketing will give you a hard time in the Q&A and… These are thoughts. They're not happening here and now. So, we can treat them like the apple-to-elephant thought—we can change them.

Pressing an acupressure point can also help to anchor your mind into the present. This next section combines our breathing techniques with acupressure point massage that you can do on yourself. It helps us to release the "stuck" energy and helps to address the associated physical and emotional discomfort. Removing the blocked energy may prevent further health issues in the body and mind.

I am quietly excited to lead you there.

Chapter 4:

Acupressure to Relieve Anxiety

Acupressure is one way to help your body fight back and balance itself in the face of the pressures of modern life. –Michael Reed Gach

"Without Qi, life is not possible," my cousin Geoff said one day as we parted. I knew he referred to energy, but it took me a while to grasp the real meaning of this two-letter word: Qi. I don't think the Oxford Dictionary quite nails it with: "The circulating life force whose existence and properties are the basis of much Chinese philosophy and medicine."

I somehow wish the lexicographer stopped after the word "force" because the words *circulate, life, and force* describe the essence of Qi or energy. Life depends on the vital force of energy that keeps everything flowing.

Our bodies run on energy. Since ancient times, Eastern healers observed that behind everything, there is energy. It is hard to explain or put into words. It's our life force, the energy that beats our hearts, moves the tides, blows the wind, shines the sun, and shifts the planets.

It is similar to how the heat of the sun is converted into electricity—the energy that keeps our modern societies moving, from traffic lights to telephones.

What Is Acupressure?

Acupressure involves using the thumb, fingertips, hand, and sometimes other tools to massage or press points on the body. By pressing identified points, blood flow increases, bringing fresh oxygen to the area. When energy flows freely, it reduces pain, and healing takes place.

You are at your desk, hard at work, when a headache sneaks up on you. What do you do? With your elbows on the desk, you probably press four fingers against each temple, the thumbs supporting the jaw bone. You inadvertently applied acupressure to ease your headache.

Chinese healers have used acupressure for many centuries. Some researchers date acupressure back to *The Yellow Emperor's Classic of Medicine*. Experts still debate when precisely this classic Chinese book was written. Some sources say the emperor Huangdi wrote it in 2,600 B.C.E. Others say it was written much later, not by a single author but by several unknown authors.

In ancient China, people only paid health practitioners once they were healthy. So, the emphasis was much more on prevention than waiting for a health problem to arise before dealing with it.

In modern medicine, the opposite happens: We go to a doctor when we are already ill and rely on doctors to address acute medical conditions.

Acupressure is not a substitute for medical care, but it can be beneficial alongside your medical treatment. It is a complementary approach to staying healthy. This technique is particularly helpful in preventative health practices and in addressing many chronic health issues.

It may improve several medical conditions and health issues, including back pain, neck pain, headache, asthma, insomnia, depression, anxiety, chronic fatigue, and more. Acupressure is similar to acupuncture but uses massage and finger pressure instead of needles.

Acupressure does not only help with physical healing. On top of physical healing, it may also help to unblock congested emotions. Sometimes we harbor disappointment, pain, or anger in our bodies for many years. We might not even realize that we still carry remnants of old sorrows. The unwritten rules of society demand that we put up a brave face and get on with life.

You might get emotional as we work through acupoints in this chapter. Don't let it worry you. Work with it and through it. Acknowledge the emotion, and even give it a name. By naming it, you add some distance between you and the emotion.

In time and with continued practice, you might feel your energy shift. And with this shift, your emotions usually follow. As you notice emotions arise, you're tuning in your conscious mind to sensations in your body. You can use a combination of the acupressure points in this section alongside exhaling deliberately through your mouth to feel a sense of relief.

Time and practice are essential. Remember, you did not get so stressed overnight. Your anxiety builds up over time. Your body needs time to unlearn its physical and emotional tension.

Athletes who recover from physical injuries find that as their bodies heal, the muscles remember and return to their former optimal strength. Your muscle memory might kick in slowly, but as the physical muscle relaxes, you may gradually feel your emotions become less intense and move.

I mentioned meridians a few times already. They are the pathways along which Qi (energy) moves in our bodies. It brings me to acupressure points along the body's meridians and how you can use them to relieve anxiety.

What Are Acupressure Points?

Our energy's movement through the meridian lines in our bodies is like a river. As a river feeds life around its banks, the energy feeds our whole body with life force energy. There are plexuses of energy throughout the body, like where a river swirls into a deeper place. This is the place where acupressure points are identified.

You can find some of these points by trying this:

- ☐ Sit on the floor and put the soles of your feet together. If that's difficult for you, you can also do this sitting in a chair with one leg over your thigh.
- ☐ Feel your ankle bone on the inside of your leg.
- ☐ Imagine someone's drawn a dotted line on the inside of your leg, along the edge of your leg bone, from the ankle to the knee.
- ☐ Now, press your thumbs up the inside of your legs along the dotted line. Do you feel some tender spots?
- ☐ Thumb press or thumb massage those points and breathe slowly and deeply.

You're actually pressing along the spleen meridian. Massaging those tender spots while slowly breathing helps to release stuck energy. And, guess what? Stress and anxiety are among the most prevalent causes of stuck energy.

Acupressure points on the body are particular spots sensitive to energy flow. When we press or massage these points, the underlying tissues stretch, and the blood and energy flow more freely.

Acupressure is safe and does not cost anything. A few minutes daily can make a significant difference. Some points are flagged as contraindicated in pregnancy or if you have a pacemaker. Otherwise, always listen to your body and amend the level of thumb pressure, or skip it. You can still achieve a shift by using a light touch, and sometimes, a soft touch can help you tune into a pulsing or another energy sensation at that point.

Some points, called trigger points, relate not only to pain in its immediate location. Think of the electrical appliances in your house. You press a light switch here, and it operates a light right over there. Sometimes you'll press an acupressure point on one part of the body and notice a sensation elsewhere.

You can do acupressure anywhere and unobtrusively, but it could be a good idea to set aside a few minutes of quiet time daily to do acupressure. Sit, or lie comfortably. Find the spot and close your eyes while you breathe deeply. It might be better to start with light pressure, increasing the firmness as you get used to it. If a pressure point feels sensitive to the touch, let it rest for a few days. Regular practice might help your physical and emotional healing.

We do not only refer to physical pain. These points may also release blocked emotions, some of which you might not even be aware of.

In the following sections, I will explain some points that may help you relieve emotional and physical pain and provide a little background on each. The names are translated from Mandarin and tell the story of their origins and purpose. The individual translations might sometimes differ slightly; therefore, I include the meridian and number combination to help you explore the specific points further.

Great Rushing, *Taichong* Liver 3 (LIV- 3)

This acupoint helps with anxiety, anger, digestion, headache, and vision.

It's fabulous for calming the mind and emotions because when you press it, all that energy from thinking, worrying, stressing, and feeling agitated just rushes down the body. So it's apt that it's called Great Rushing.

Maybe you're sitting at your desk, in a meeting, on a video phone, or at a restaurant. And, maybe, you start to feel stressed or anxious. Perhaps you feel that the conversation isn't going too well, you think you've said something to offend the other person, or you're just feeling nervous.

Or, maybe you want to unwind at home after a stressful day. Here's what you can do. Try practicing it now.

- ☐ It is located on the top of the foot, between the big and second toe.

- Slip your right shoe off.

- With your right heel, press, and massage into the LIV-3 point between the big toe and the next toe.

- Slow your breathing.

- Take a few slow breaths as you stimulate each point. The breath resets the nervous system, making acupressure more effective. You can also press the point in various ways: thumb, finger massage, pressing the point, tapping your fingers, or tapping with your fist.

- If you're relaxing at home, do this for about a minute. Do what you can wherever you are.

- Repeat with the other foot.

- Now, this is important: Take a moment to notice the shift inside you. Often, it can be quite subtle, especially at first. Do you feel a little calmer? Less agitated? Just notice, like you're observing yourself.

- If you catch yourself analyzing the degree to which you've shifted, you've pinged out of observation mode into that ever-thinking and often self-critical mind. Just take a breath, and try not to judge!

Inner Pass, Pericardium 6 (P-6)

It helps with emotional protection, anxiety, and nausea. Doctors often recommend applying pressure to P-6 for patients who are nauseous after surgery. Some cancer patients also find this helpful point to reduce nausea during chemotherapy.

The Chinese name is *Neiguan*, which translates into Inner Pass.

The pericardium is a protective membrane around the heart. In Chinese medicine, the pericardium energy pathway and the acupoints along it help to protect the heart itself. They also protect the heart's energy, which we know as emotions. They say that when the heart energy (the fire element) is depleted, we feel the need to be over-busy, hasty, and impatient. When the heart's energy is in balance, we return to our default, a frequency of happiness, joy, love, and compassion.

- ☐ It is located on the inside of the wrist, about three fingers down. It is between the tendons, which feel a bit like elastic bands.

- ☐ Hold your hand with your palm facing you.

- ☐ Place three fingers of your other hand across the wrist crease at the base of the palm.

- ☐ The point is three finger widths along the wrist crease.

- ☐ Press your thumb down gently, feeling the two tendons running down your arm.

- ☐ Hold and repeat several times.

- ☐ Change to the other wrist and repeat the process.

Great Mound, Pericardium 7 (P-7)

This helps with anxiety, irritability, relationships, heart palpitations, and insomnia.

This acupoint is close to the Inner Pass. Interestingly, this point has several other names: Daling, Heart Governor, Great Hill, Great Plateau, and Ghost Heart. The variety of names reflects the Great Mound's popularity in Eastern healing practices. Eastern healers believe the waste from the spleen accumulates here, thus, forming a mound. By pressing or massaging, Qi can flow freely, releasing waste.

- ☐ It is located between the tendons in the middle of the wrist crease.

- ☐ Rest your forearm palm facing upward on a firm surface.

- [ ] Find P7 in the middle of the wrist crease between the tendons.

- [ ] Put the thumb of your other hand on the spot. You can also use the index finger.

- [ ] Press gently, or more firmly, down to best suit you until you feel the tendons.

- [ ] Massage in small circles without lifting the thumb or finger from the skin. You can also apply an up-and-down movement, pressuring firmly.

- [ ] Continue for about two minutes, breathing deeply.

- [ ] Repeat with opposite hands.

Palace of Toil, Pericardium 8 (P-8)

P-8 helps with anxiety, nervous tension, and tightness in the chest.

We shake hands touching this point and often communicate by gesturing with our hands. You may have noticed how people from different religions and spiritual movements bless each other with an open palm. The open palm has spiritual meaning in many groups. In Eastern tradition, healers use their palms to expand their life-force energy to another person. No wonder the Palace of Toil is considered a powerful acupoint in healing our hearts and sorrows.

I'll give you two ways to apply pressure to P-8 so you can choose what suits you best.

- [ ] It is in the middle of the palm, where the ring finger's tip comes to rest when making a fist.

- [ ] Hold both hands in front of you, palms facing you.

- [ ] Put one hand on the other.

☐ Bring the thumb of the bottom hand to the center of the top hand.

☐ Move the thumb in tiny circles.

☐ Put your attention here. Gently concentrate on the point and the slight movement.

Gushing Spring, Kidney 1 (K-1)

Kidney 1 helps with anxiety, nervous tension, tightness in the chest, and insomnia. If you, like so many of us, find the mind racing at bedtime, applying acupressure to Kidney 1 may help calm the mind.

Gushing Spring, on the soles of the feet, is the lowest acupoint. Therefore, activating this point stimulates the body to release excess energy downward, away from our head and mind. Sometimes our daily challenges, rushing from one task to another, get too much. Our hearts and kidneys get out of balance, and our minds become overactive.

This point brings the energy down the body so that the busy mind can calm. Firm pressure at this point gathers all the excess energy and lets it flow, as water flows from a spring.

I'll show you different ways to sit and also a few techniques to add if you want to activate the energy flow more vigorously.

It is located on the foot sole between the bones of the second and third toes. If you draw a line from the base of the second toe to the heel, the point is about one-third down from the second toe's base. If you flex all your toes inward, K-1 is in the dip.

☐ Sit on a solid surface.

☐ Seated, you can stretch out one leg, swing the other leg over, and firmly grab the target foot with your hand. Use the thumb of the free hand to apply pressure while breathing slowly and deeply.

☐ You could also sit cross-legged, swing the arm under one of your legs and lift it toward your chest. Now grab the toes with your hand and use the free hand for the massage.

☐ Whichever way you use to grab hold of the foot, press firmly onto the acupoint for half a minute while breathing slowly and deeply.

☐ Massage the point with your thumb in small circles while breathing slowly and deeply.

☐ If you find it difficult to reach, here is another clever way. Use a tennis ball or a rolled-up sock and roll it underneath the foot to stimulate the point.

☐ If you feel energetic, you can use two additional techniques.

  o Use your fist and start knocking your foot sole while holding the foot firmly with the other hand. It invigorates the body and gets the energy flowing.

  o Then, start slapping the foot sole rhythmically with the free hand. The slapping continues to signal the upper body to release excess energy.

☐ Return to a cross legged position with both feet on the floor.

☐ Lean forward and grab a foot in each hand.

☐ Return to pressing K-1, but consciously combine your breathing with your body movements.

☐ Lean slightly back and breathe in while holding the thumbs on the acupoint.

☐ Lean forward while breathing out and push the thumbs into the acupoint using your body weight to enforce the pressure while breathing slowly and deeply.

You can do a more advanced technique if you are fit. Always listen to your body and do what is comfortable for you on the day.

- [ ] In the same position, cross-legged and holding on to the feet with the thumbs on K-1, breathe in and roll back.

- [ ] Roll forward while breathing out.

- [ ] Pause for a second and press your body weight into the acupoints more actively.

- [ ] Repeat and use your breath to continue rolling.

Spirit Gate, Heart Meridian Point 7 (H-7)

Pressure to the Spirit Gate helps with anxiety, insomnia, regaining emotional balance, heart palpitations, motion sickness, and depression.

Pressure on this point unlocks the gate that blocks your energy. You can do this in the privacy of your home as part of your regular program. But stimulating the Spirit Gate is easy to do unobtrusively at the office or commuting. This point helps balance emotional energy, especially in relationships.

- [ ] It is located in the crease of the wrist. Draw an imaginary line from the space between your ring and little finger to the wrist crease.

- [ ] Hold your hand with the palm facing you.

- [ ] Firmly grab your wrist with your other thumb on the spot.

- [ ] Apply mild but firm pressure for up to 30 seconds.

- [ ] Massage with thumb circles and press the point gently for about 30 seconds to a minute on each hand.

Lesser Palace, Heart Point 8 (H-8)

Heart 8 helps with anxiety, insomnia, emotional balance, fear, and sadness. It also addresses heart palpitations, chest pain, difficulty urinating, bed wetting, and pinky pain.

In traditional Chinese medicine, the heart influences the entire body—physically and emotionally. Chinese emperors were called supreme rulers and lived in grand palaces through the ages. Eastern philosophers called the human heart the Lesser Palace, a place to rest and revitalize out of respect for their emperors. When emotionally overwrought and exhausted, we can revive the spirit by returning to the heart.

- ☐ To find Heart 8's location, lie your hand flat with your palm facing you. Make a loose fist and bend the pinky so that its tip touches the palm. It is the Lesser Palace point.

- ☐ Hold the hand, palm facing you.

- ☐ With the thumb from your other hand, press firmly for a moment and release. Breathe slowly and relax.

- ☐ Repeat for about a minute, breathing slowly and deeply.

- ☐ Reverse hands and repeat.

Grandfather Grandson, Spleen 4 (SP-4)

Spleen 4 helps with emotional balance, calms the heart's energy, and helps you feel grounded. Eastern healers often use Spleen 4 with other acupoints because of its strong influence on emotions. It is especially powerful when used with acupoints relevant to the abdomen and heart.

The name—Grandfather Grandson—tells the multi-layered history of this acupoint and gives some insight into the history of traditional Chinese medicine. The Chinese name is *Gongsun*, the family name of the legendary emperor and founder of Taoism and Chinese medicine.

The English version, Grandfather Grandson, hints at its eternal importance in the human body.

- It is located in the arch of the foot. An easy way to find Spleen Point 4 is to start at the side of the big toe and move your finger down along the outer edge, over the bump. You have now arrived at Spleen 3. Carry on for about an inch along the bone to its base to find Spleen 4. Spleen points 3 and 4 are in the valley between the bone and muscle that run along the length of the foot toward the heel.

- Rest your foot on a flat surface like your bed, with the arch facing you.

- Thumb press and massage this point.

- Massage along the whole of the arch toward the ankle. In this way, you massage Spleen 3 and 4.

- Remember to press firmly. But listen to your body and modify the pressure to suit you. Breathe deep and slow.

- Massage for about a minute on each foot.

Three Yin Intersection, *Sanyinjiao* Spleen 6 (SP-6)

*This point is not recommended for pregnant women.

This point helps for emotional balance and to calm heart energy. But Spleen 6 also helps with many physical ailments.

Spleen 6 is the junction point of the liver, spleen, and kidney meridians. No wonder it is so versatile. On this point, acupressure addresses a variety of physical and emotional conditions relating to these three organs. From chapter two, we know that stress and anxiety are considered to be an imbalance of liver and kidney energy and that mental anxiety is associated with spleen energy.

- It is located about four fingers above the inner ankle—feel for a tender spot.

- ☐ Swing one leg over the other.

- ☐ Use your hand from the same side as the leg you are pressing.

- ☐ Grasp your leg and apply pressure with your thumb for a few seconds.

- ☐ Release to light pressure, apply medium pressure, then light pressure.

- ☐ Continue in this way for about a minute on each foot, breathing slowly and deeply.

These are just a few of the acupressure points you can use. If you'd like to try some more, I recommend Michael Reed Gach's book, Acupressure's Potent Points (1990). As well as acupressure, we can use Qigong exercises to circulate energy around the body. There are some great exercises for anxiety relief in the next chapter.

Chapter 5:

Qigong for Anxiety

Qigong is more than a set of exercises; it is an attitude that works to restructure one's perspective on life, leading to balance and harmony with the world around us.
–Francesco Garri Garripoli

What is Qigong?

Qigong is pronounced "Chee-gong", which means "energy work." Qi means energy, and gong means work skillfully. It is the basic exercise system in Eastern tradition with calming, meditative movements for relaxation and mental clarity. It preserves physical health and builds spiritual strength. If we regularly do Qigong exercises, our bodies automatically build up energy reserves for those unforeseen and challenging events that cross our paths.

Traditional Chinese medicine considers our physical ailments connected to our emotional states. Eastern healers say fear, agitation, and irritability cause our anxiety. The muscles tense up in preparation for danger, consequently blocking the body's natural energy flow. We need this energy to do what we want to do in our lives. Our impatient lifestyle makes us feel wired and tired. We hold our nervous system in red-alert mode and restrict blood flow and energy needed to mend and replenish our cells.

Interestingly, ancient Mandarin did not have a direct translation for the word "anxiety." However, related symptoms like insomnia, overthinking, and worrying are directly linked to fire energy in the heart.

Traditional Chinese philosophy recognizes five elements. in the body: fire, water, earth, wood, and metal. Each element is connected to a specific organ. When a particular element becomes unbalanced in the organ, the body and the emotions are affected.

The heart rules our blood circulation, and it houses our spirit. When our heart's fire energy is unbalanced, we are anxious, agitated, and have difficulty sleeping. Keeping the fire energy balanced helps to combat anxiety and cultivate the higher vibrations of joy, love, happiness, and compassion. Qigong is ideal for opening the energy pathways and allowing energy to flow freely.

In Chinese medicine, the spleen represents the earth element. The spleen filters blood, helps defend the body against pathogens, and plays a role in transporting fluids around the body.

If the spleen meridian is blocked, the body gets out of sync and is unbalanced. The result is mental anxiety, repetitive thoughts, overthinking, worry, and mind fog. When we strengthen spleen energy, we can be more grounded and centered, cultivate stability, an open mind, clear thinking, intuition, and develop insight.

The lungs are the center of our respiration system, regulating oxygen distribution and removing carbon dioxide. We know the adverse physical symptoms such as shortness of breath, fatigue, and allergies that a lack of fresh oxygen causes. In Eastern tradition, the lungs are also connected with emotions such as depression and anxiety. By strengthening lung function, our physical health improves, but with the lungs' metal energy, we can cultivate courage and positivity.

The liver stores blood and regulates smooth blood flow and bile secretion. Chinese healers believe the liver's wood energy is connected to anger, frustration, agitation, and stress. The kidneys also remove waste from the body, and Chinese healers connect gloomy emotions such as fear, weak willpower, insecurity, and wanting to isolate yourself from others with the kidneys. By freeing the energy pathways to the kidneys, their water energy can bring peace and calm.

Qigong practices can help to unblock the energy pathways in the body. As the energy flows, our anxiety levels drop, we are more relaxed, and emotional and physical healing may occur. Qigong practices use breath, movement, focus, posture, and relaxation—elements vital to our emotional and physical health. Thus, whatever your needs, genetics, age, or lifestyle, Qigong practices can help you relax and heal.

Over the last few years, Qigong has become a lifestyle for me. It is not an exercise program or something I do now and then when I have time. It is an integral part of my life, and I make time for it. Although Qigong exercises are gentle and, on the surface, unassuming, they changed my life for the better.

I suffered from excess nervous energy for a long time. Nervous energy is not bad in itself. It can help us in a dangerous situation but, unfortunately, also keep us awake at night. My daily Qigong routine helps to restore harmony in my body and mind, even during stressful times. "Balance" is a key concept in Qigong, and when life gets rushed, I slip away to do a few Qigong practices.

Qigong's movements are gentle breathing, stretching, and mindfulness. They helped me to calm my mind, clear my energy pathways, and lessen my anxiety.

In the previous chapter, I guided you to several acupressure points that may help relieve anxiety. Through Qigong, you can unblock the energy flow throughout the body, an essential step in reducing anxiety.

Qigong is for everyone—you don't have to be young and fit. Qigong exercises are gentle, and I will lead you gradually into the basic stances. You then can choose practices that suit your physical, mental, and emotional needs.

Basic Qigong Principles

It is important not to rush any movement or breathing. Inhale deeply, exhale slowly and let your focus go with the breath and the movement. Also, keep the knees slightly bent, as it helps keep the spine aligned and the body relaxed.

We start with wave breathing, as this practice illustrates the slow flow of movement, breath, and focus while the body is relaxed and the spine aligned.

Wave Breathing for Inner Calm

In the previous chapter, I introduced you to wave breathing to help you sleep. The version I'll illustrate here harmonizes the head, heart, and body for inner calm. It is one of the basic but most potent Qigong practices. We tend to underuse our lungs, and the lungs' flexibility is a positive indicator of longevity. This practice encourages us to use the lungs more effectively.

- ☐ Stand with knees slightly bent.

- ☐ Let's do wave breathing with one hand on the chest and the other on the belly. Remember, you are doing slow breathing. Do not rush; savor every moment by focusing on your breath.

- ☐ Inhale through your nose, fill the belly, the ribs, and the chest, and exhale through the nose as you relax the chest, then the ribs, then the belly.

- ☐ Breathe in deeply to bring new energy into the body.

- ☐ Exhale to rid the body of old stale energy.

We are now extending the waves and stretching the breath mechanics a little bit.

- ☐ Bring your hands over your elbows and hold them there, forming a circle with your arms.

- ☐ Inhale, bringing your arms up and overhead.

- ☐ Exhale and come down nice and slow.

- ☐ Switch hands so that the outside one comes in.

- Inhale, drifting your arms up, exhale nice and slow, floating them down. We are stretching through the ribs, the intercostal muscles, and the diaphragm, bringing more flexibility into the mechanics of the breath.

- Relax your arms down the sides.

We are now entering a new phase of wave breathing. This exercise is called Single Hand Waterfall. We bring some energy down the conception vessel (the energy path down the front of your body), and we join the energy centers along this meridian—the energy from the mid-eye between the brows, mind, heart, solar plexus, and belly. Breathe deeply for the duration of the movement.

Single Hand Waterfall

- Before we start, take a look at your hand. The V-shape between the thumb and the first finger is called the tiger's mouth. We align the tiger's mouth to the central energy channel running down the front body.

- With your palm facing up, keep your right hand under your belly, with your knees soft and slightly bent. Relax your shoulders and relax your hips.

- Bring your left hip and your left shoulder slightly forward. With your wrist relaxed, let your left-hand float up and hover the tiger's mouth over the mid-eye. Let your focus follow the movement and your breath.

- As the tiger's mouth comes to the mid-eye, let it drift down the center front line while you exhale slowly. Bend your knees slightly and sink into the movement. Your concentration follows the direction of the energy down.

- Change hands. Your left hand comes to your belly, palm facing up.

- Bring the right hip and the right shoulder forward.

- Inhale deeply and with your right wrist relaxed, let your hand float up and drift down while you breathe in and then out.

- ☐ Your focus stays on the breath and the movement.

- ☐ Repeat for about two to three minutes.

Now for the next phase of this practice. This exercise is called Pulling down the Heavens. It brings excess energy down from our busy minds into the belly, so it's very calming.

Pulling down the Heavens

- ☐ Remember, you breathe slowly, and the body is relaxed.

- ☐ Stand with feet shoulder-width apart, knees relaxed.

- ☐ When you inhale, float your arms up at the sides, gathering the energy you want to draw in.

- ☐ At the top, hold your hands over your head, palm over palm, but not touching.

- ☐ Exhale and move your hands down the front line, bringing the energy into the belly.

- ☐ Repeat for about two minutes. Alternate which hand goes on top. Palm over palm, move the energy down smooth and flowing. You bring energy to the belly and contain it there.

Now for a bit of variation:

- ☐ Next time, when your hands reach your belly, cross the wrists and touch the thumb and first finger together to form two circles.

- ☐ The next movement is almost like you are going to pull a belt tighter. Pull your elbows back and pull the belt as you inhale.

- ☐ Exhale and release your hands to the sides.

- ☐ Inhale and open your arms, drifting them upward. Exhale, palm over palm, drifting your hands down along the conception vessel.

- ☐ Inhale as you cross the wrists, and pull the belt. Exhale as you relax your arms down.

- ☐ Repeat this movement for about two minutes.

And to close down, this exercise is called Bamboo in the Wind.

- ☐ Bring your feet together and hold your palms over your belly.

- ☐ Relax behind your knees, under your feet, and your shoulders.

- ☐ Breathe deep and slow.

- ☐ You might find yourself rocking and swaying a little like bamboo in the wind as you relax. Just go with the flow and let the energy guide you.

Water Waves

Water waves brings the energy down to the body and center it in the belly. It is guaranteed to let you feel free as a young child. This fun practice has a deeper purpose, though. It may help you feel calmer and more grounded.

- ☐ Stand feet shoulder-width apart, knees softly bent.

- ☐ Close your eyes, or keep them open, whichever works best for you.

- ☐ Turn your hips left and right while your arms trail around you. Your arms move as if you are in a pool of water, making ripple circles around you.

- ☐ Relax your shoulders and breathe slowly while you turn from your center, trailing the arms for about two minutes.

☐ Put your mind to your feet and hips and breath, feeling the air through your fingertips.

Clearing Heavy Energy

Right in the center of the chest, on the sternum (breastbone), is the heart center, where emotional energy is gathered. This exercise opens the chest and the area between the shoulder blades. It releases emotional energy from the heart—anything weighing heavily on your heart. This practice is similar to water waves, but the arms are at shoulder height.

☐ Stand with the feet shoulder width.

☐ Inhale as you raise your arms to shoulder height.

☐ Exhale through your mouth as you bend your knees, drop your arms, and swing your right arm across in front of your body, left arm behind. You're twisting to look left.

☐ Then inhale as you swing your arms up and open at shoulder height, your body facing forward.

☐ Exhale as you bend your knees, twist, look right, and let your left arm swing in front and your right arm behind you.

☐ Repeat for about two minutes.

Releasing Emotional Energy That We No Longer Need

This practice is ideal for relieving tension and is easy to do. Remember, the chest contains the heart center, where we sometimes hold blocked emotional energy. In the following practice, you will learn more about sound breathing, but this Tarzan-like technique is an excellent introduction to the healing properties of sound.

☐ Make fists and knock up and down your sternum. It causes vibrations on the fascia in the chest, like you're loosening the pent-up emotions.

- Repeat knocking on the chest, but this time, make an HAAA sound when you exhale. Have the intention of letting go of any emotional energy that no longer serves you.

- Repeat for a minute or so.

- I hope you feel more relaxed after this practice.

Healing Sounds

Most of us agree: Singing is good for the soul. Like singing, sometimes Qigong also uses sound breathing that can have several physical and emotional benefits. In Mandarin, the words for medicine and sound are very similar: *Yao* and *Yue*.

Qigong has a set of healing sounds that are particularly good for when we recover from trauma, illness, or an operation. Singing and sound breathing are both aerobic activities and increase the oxygen flow in the bloodstream. Healing sounds can strengthen the body's ability to heal.

Each of the Qigong healing sounds is connected to a specific organ pair. Sound is concentrated energy that vibrates through the body like a tuning fork. The sounds we use are thought to correspond to the healthiest frequency of each organ and its related body system. When we exhale making these sounds, the corresponding organs release excess energy and toxins.

Our health can benefit by using slow breathing and sound together. Slow breathing resets the nervous system so the body can regenerate the cells.

Remember, sound breathing and singing are based on the same principles. And music is part of life; it speaks to our emotions and adds value to our lives. You can try sound breathing and notice if you feel more comfortable in yourself when you have completed it.

The following practice is good to do in the shower if you feel self-conscious. First, try a whispering sound. Then go softer and still softer until you make the shape with your mouth. Here's the trick: Use your mind to locate the sound as if it's happening inside the organ.

Organs and Healing Sounds

- You can make healing sounds while sitting, lying, or standing.

- Inhale soft and slow through your nose.

  o Exhale with the sound SSS for healthy lung energy.

- Inhale soft and slow through your nose.

  o Exhale with the sound CHWOO for healthy kidney energy.

- Inhale soft and slow through your nose.

  o Exhale with the sound SSHH for healthy liver energy.

- Inhale soft and slow through your nose.

  o Exhale with the sound HAAA for healthy heart energy.

- Inhale soft and slow through your nose.

  o Exhale with the sound HAAW for healthy spleen energy.

- Inhale soft and slow through your nose.

  o Exhale with the sound HEEE for overall balance and health. *Triple Warmer energy.

- Repeat this set three to ten times, morning and evening. Do more if you want to.

  *The Triple Warmer harmonizes the head, heart, and body.

Pebble in the Pond

You have heard it so often, maybe even said it yourself: gut feeling. Your gut is like a second brain because of the neurological activity in the belly. Let the wisdom of the body—the belly and earth center—speak to your mind.

- ☐ Stand feet shoulder-width apart. Relax knees, shoulders, and tailbone.

- ☐ Slowly breathe into the belly. It expands as you breathe in and relaxes as you breathe out.

- ☐ Take a couple of slow breaths in and out through the nose.

- ☐ Exhale, gliding your hips back a little bit.

- ☐ As you do this and relax your shoulders, your arms float up automatically.

- ☐ Inhale while you bend your knees a little bit and stand tall, as your arms come in toward your belly, drawing the energy into the center.

- ☐ Repeat in a slow and relaxed way for two to three minutes.

Now you do the second stage of Pebble in the Pond, which is an excellent way to clear the mind.

- ☐ Have your left-hand palm up under your belly and your right palm down a few inches above your left hand.

- ☐ Send your right hand out toward your left and circle it forward and right like it's skimming across a pond, sending positive energy from you out to the world.

- ☐ Bring your right hand back to the center, bringing the positive energy back to you. Stand tall.

- ☐ Turn your left hand, palm facing down, and circle it forward.

☐ Return the left hand back to the belly center, bringing positive energy back to your center.

☐ Your hands move slowly, like through water, across the body to your right, circle forward in front of you, and back round the body.

☐ Repeat for two to three minutes.

☐ Bring the palms to the belly and take a few relaxed breaths.

You can integrate these short exercises anytime into your day. When you can, doing one or two regular Qigong classes every week can also be good for building your energy and releasing energy that no longer serves you.

These exercises are from classes at LessStressMoreEnergy.com and are based on Lee Holden's approach to Qigong.

Chapter 6:

A Shift in Me Creates a Shift in You

If you restore balance in your own self, you will be contributing immensely to the healing of the world. —Deepak Chopra

Have you noticed how some people are easy to be around, and others make you feel out of balance? You might have been in a situation where you have been uncomfortable with a particular person.

In this chapter, we'll build on some of the techniques we've been practicing. We take it a step further to cultivate protective energy around us and guide, direct and project our positive energy to others.

We have a measurable energy field. Like the earth has gravity, our personal energy field is invisible. Modern science can measure the unique signature of our heart, muscles, and brain via highly advanced systems: electrocardiography (ECG), electromyography (EMG), and electroencephalography (EEG). As you practice the techniques in this book, you might notice a shift in how you feel and a change in how people behave around you. Other people can sense it consciously or subconsciously. Our mental and emotional energy takes shape in our bodies.

Try raising your eyebrows and feeling sad. It's not possible! When we feel depressed or sad, we hunch our chest. In Chinese medicine, strengthening the lung energy not only benefits the respiratory and immune systems. It also sets your lung frequency to healthier levels, which results in confidence and inspiration. So, as you practice, your physiology is changed.

The cellular biologist Dr. Bruce Lipton and others have concluded from a body of research that while our DNA provides a predisposition, it is our perceptions (mind) and responses (emotions) that determine whether or not the reactions in our DNA are triggered.

Acquired Qi

My Qigong teacher calls it "acquired Qi," where we are affected by other people's energy, positive or negative. Unfortunately, we detect other people's negativity very quickly. When they are snappy with us, we pick it up. The negativity snowballs: We feel anxious, stressed, and unhappy, and in turn, people around us pick up on our bad moods.

We all know people who make you feel drained or anxious by their mere presence. It's because you subconsciously tune into their frequency and vibrate along with them. If your thoughts attach and your mind starts to create a pessimistic movie repeatedly, this gloomy energy may become lodged in you. This negativity may also get stuck in your energy field from listening to the news or negative conversations. It could even be negativity from your childhood.

The approaches in this book can strengthen your energy and help you release someone or something else's negative Qi. You return to your true, authentic, and original energy when you release the past or worry about the future. You feel lighter without the acquired energy from others. You might feel more yourself, but the people around you also start to notice that they feel good around you.

Here is a short trick to improve rapport next time you are with people. Notice their breathing. Do they breathe in the chest, quick and shallow? This gives us a clue as to how they are feeling. When people talk, they exhale. As they start talking, synchronize your exhale to theirs. Try this and feel how the energy in the room becomes more harmonious.

Quick Trick to Minimize Negative Energy 1

Here is another quick way to reduce the impact of someone's negative energy and prevent it from attaching to you.

☐ If you sense persistent negative energy, check out the other person's breathing unobtrusively. Deliberately slow down your breathing.

□ By changing your breath rate, you can start to feel dislodged from the other person's negative frequency. By observing rather than taking on their energy, you'll help to maintain inner balance.

Slow breathing into your belly can help you feel more grounded, and your body is less like a sponge lapping up negativity from around you.

As we inhale, we're drawing in energy from nature and the people around us. As we exhale, we send our energy out into our surroundings. Our energy and the energy around us are the same. The Taoists refer to the energy around us as The Sea Of Qi. Quantum Physics refers to it as the quantum field. Energy manifests in different forms. It may be invisible, but like Wi-Fi, we know it's still there.

Remember, energy is vibrations, and according to the laws of quantum physics, we are all interconnected. You can consciously prevent the negative energy around you from affecting your energy. So remember, small shifts in your own mind can change how you react to the negativity around you.

Just as you experience somebody's negativity exhausting you and robbing you of your vitality, you can try the reverse. As you begin to cultivate healthier, positive energy, other people may be able to feel it. It's like throwing a pebble in the pond, which ripples outward.

Quick Trick to Minimize Negative Energy 2

So, let's check in to the quick breathing technique above.

□ You have checked out the person's breathing rate and slowed yours down to feel calm and grounded.

□ Notice the other person; just observe and notice their emotions and how they feel without judgment.

□ Continued deep breathing helps you to remain calm. You create distance between yourself and the other person by engaging your conscious attention.

☐ You can also drop a word into your exhale without speaking out loud. A positive word, like "calm" or "peace." It's like the vibration of that word is a pebble that you are dropping into the sea of Qi.

☐ Check-in with how you feel. Notice that you have moved your energy from agitated to calm. Observe the other person's breathing, and notice if there's a shift.

Quick Trick to Help Get Rid of Negative Energy or Toxins

Now for some practice cleaning yourself of negative energy from people or the environment lodged inside you.

☐ Pat your right palm down the inside of your left arm from the front of the shoulder down to the wrist. It is where the heart and pericardium energy meridians go, so you're activating energy there.

☐ Grasp the wrist firmly. Then, firmly brush off across the left palm as you exhale through the mouth, releasing energy you no longer want, including other people's energy.

☐ Repeat several times on each side.

Sometimes, it can feel like we just want to press the reset button and return to being ourselves before all the stress. Here's another technique I've found useful. It's based on a neuro-linguistic programming (NLP) approach.

Technique to Clear Your Mind

☐ Breathe deeply, eyes closed, and gently relax each part of your body, neck, jaw, and shoulders. Take your mind all the way through, relaxing each part until you reach your toes. Take another breath, hold it for a second, and then exhale.

☐ See the incident or person that causes your anxiety. Picture whatever makes you anxious, like it's on a movie screen.

- ☐ Now put a frame around the picture. Is the frame in place?

- ☐ Is there noise or sound? Can you hear voices? How loud is the sound? Give it a number out of 10.

- ☐ Turn the volume down in your mind. What number is the sound now?

- ☐ Are there things or people moving around, or is your picture still? If there is some activity, make it still.

- ☐ If there are colors, change them to black and white.

- ☐ How intense are the feelings or sensations in this picture? Turn the intensity down from ten to a lower number.

- ☐ Take your picture and half it in size. Half again, and again.

- ☐ Move the picture down to the bottom right of your screen.

- ☐ Half it again and again until it is just a dot. Eventually, notice it is gone.

If you're interested in finding out more about NLP, try Ali Campbell's book, *NLP made easy* (2015).

The Shift in Me

I gradually became aware of the subtle shift in my emotions as I implemented breathwork in my daily life. I managed better at work as I increasingly managed to control my anxiety.

However, I had a long way to go. I dreaded the monthly meetings with our biggest client. I was uncomfortable with Fred, the client's marketing manager. He was loud and took over every meeting. In my opinion, he was arrogant, and when he didn't get his way, it sometimes bordered on being rude.

The senior partner asked me to chair the meeting a day before the monthly meeting. "And don't let Fred hijack the meeting," he said before ending the call. I felt sick when I met Geoff for a coffee later that day. Geoff listened to my ranting and smiled. "You can allow this guy to drain your energy, ruin the meeting, or turn the situation around."

"In times of stress, it helps me to remember that we are one with the surrounding universe," Geoff explained. "I first try to move the negative energy in my mind down to the earth. As you know, when you breathe slowly, your brain calms, and you lift your emotion. And this is the wonder of Qi. You may also spread your positive energy to others."

Although I heard Geoff's words, I was still skeptical. Quantum physics is one thing, but the interconnectedness of energy in a lawyers' meeting? It was a bit much.

Still, as I shared in Chapter 1, Geoff played a role in my emotional development. He was present in one of my earliest childhood memories and popped up again in my current crisis. As a toddler, I refused his invitation to play ball, which set the tone for most of my life. I was determined not to pass up another opportunity to play ball.

I so often absorbed negative energy from around me. It might be because Geoff is right: The entire universe is interconnected, and ultimately Fred's arrogance can deplete my energy, or could it be that my newfound calm can shift Fred's energy?

Deeply puzzled, I said goodbye to Geoff. Was this science? Eastern philosophy? Given the positive shift in my emotions, I was willing to give it a go.

This is what happened at the meeting the next day:

I kept breathing into my belly while people took their seats. Fred entered laughing and joking, ignoring my effort to start the meeting on time.

I felt a suffocating tightness in my chest but went to my breath for relief. I did some box breathing: inhale for four, hold for four and exhale for four while observing Fred. Sure enough, just pacing my breath gave me a little reprieve, and I remembered Geoff's words about observing, not judging. I looked at the man across from me and saw him as he was in his chair. He seemed shorter than I remembered, not as threatening.

For the first time, I noticed his voice went a few octaves higher as he spoke loudly and gestured wildly. He laughed at his own jokes. Then it clicked—Fred was nervous. His breath was shallow, and his eyes darted around as if looking for support.

I deliberately lengthened my exhale, as Geoff recommended. By focusing on my breathing, my mind calmed. Without consciously deciding the moment was right, I sent Fred a wordless message: "It's OK. Be calm. It's OK."

I felt a sense of relief, even peace, as my unspoken words traveled across the table. I visualized the message softly, vibrating with positive energy. The meeting took off, and I repeated my message to Fred several times. It came naturally, and I was intensely grateful to share my newfound positivity with Fred and the world. It was as if my emotions moved outward, and I sensed the atmosphere become lighter.

Fred frowned slightly as if puzzled. He did not interrupt the speakers as he previously had done. He listened attentively, and several people who rarely spoke in meetings made valuable comments. It was a fruitful discussion, and we ended the session on time.

Did Fred sense the positive energy I had projected on him? I will never know, but as we walked to the lift, I kept sending him thoughts: "You're OK. You're doing fine."

I was proud and grateful that the meeting went well. More importantly, I was overjoyed as I discovered I actually liked my job. I enjoyed being a lawyer. I liked my life.

We cannot always control our circumstances. Sometimes, life happens, and you might feel the need to protect yourself. Maybe you feel particularly vulnerable; perhaps you have experienced intense loss.

When you need extra protection, Qigong and similar techniques may help you, whatever your situation.

Protecting Yourself

Wei Qi is the energy field you can build around you to guard against negative energy affecting you. The earth's energy field is gravity. Like the earth, we have our own energy field, which these practices may help to strengthen.

When you are particularly stressed, Taoists say that the emotional fire in your heart is out of balance, and the heat rises to the head, making the mind agitated. With your energy depleted, your Wei Qi becomes weaker, making you more susceptible to negativity from someone else.

Here, I give you two practices to strengthen your Qi so you can feel safe and grounded throughout your day. The first practice stimulates two acupressure points in the body that boost the immune system, lessen anxiety, and restore balance. Their names tell it all: Outer Gate and Inner Gate.

Build Protective Energy: Wei Chi

☐ Stand with feet shoulder-width and breathe deeply.

☐ Lift your forearms and cross your wrists at approximately chest height.

☐ Cross your wrists at the point where your watch strap would be, palms facing you. If you want to make sure:

   ○ Outer gate *Waiguan*—On the outer arm, the point (TW-5) is three fingers from the wrist crease.

   ○ Inner gate *Neiguan*—On the inner arm, the point (P-6) is three fingers from the wrist crease. The wrists are not quite touching.

☐ Exhale and part hands, palms facing, as if you're clearing away anything weighing heavy on your heart. Then float your arms down your sides, palms facing the earth.

☐ Inhale, lifting your arms slowly, crossing them at the chest.

☐ Send the energy you have released down to the earth.

☐ Feel the positive energy you have cultivated in the palms of your hands. Imagine a golden light from your palms spreading over your shoulders, round your back, and then surrounding you: at your sides, above, below, and in front.

☐ In your mind, say to yourself, "I am safe and protected."

☐ Then bring your hands to your belly, hook your thumbs and hold your energy in the belly where it anchors you firmly to the earth.

There are different variations of this practice. Give one of them a try when you feel threatened or need protection.

Wei Qi Against Energy Thieves

Sit, or stand for this practice, as long as you are comfortable. We start with a silent meditation but will go over into a moving meditation. The following practice can be helpful if you want to shield yourself from feeling drained and depleted by some people. In a quiet place, sitting or standing comfortably, close your eyes.

☐ With your mouth closed, rest the tip of your tongue just behind the upper teeth.

☐ Begin with abdominal breathing through your nose, letting the belly expand and relax as you breathe deeply.

☐ Feel the flow of breath in your body and the relaxing effect in your body and settling the mind.

When you feel harmony in your breathing and mind, we continue with a short meditation using the five main organs. In the traditional five element theory, organs are associated with aspects of nature and colors on the color light spectrum. Each organ is associated with a color matching the organ's optimal health frequency. It also helps us visualize Qi's flow. We use the breath to activate the energy of the organs, allowing their Qi to move beyond the body to form a shield around us.

- ☐ Continue deep belly breathing and visualize the top of the head as a door opening to the sky.

- ☐ Follow the light in your mind's eye as it flows down the body and settles in the abdomen. The fresh Qi keeps flowing in from above, pouring into your body.

- ☐ Now move your mind to your spleen (the Earth Element). Visualize a yellow light coming up from the earth into the left side of your body. The yellow light securely connects you to the earth and stabilizes your body and mind.

- ☐ The light descending from the universe and the yellow light from the earth mix in your belly, behind and a little below your navel, your body center. When your mind goes there, your energy follows, helping you to feel centered, grounded, and in touch with the stability of the earth.

- ☐ Remember to continue breathing slowly and deeply.

- ☐ Move your mind to your kidneys (the Water Element) at the back. Visualize the kidneys opening and releasing their Qi in a sparkling blue like the ocean, bringing peace and tranquility.

- ☐ Remember to continue breathing slowly and deeply, seeing the kidney Qi flowing around your back body in a protective layer.

- ☐ Move your mind to your heart (the Fire Element), the protection center. Visualize the heart opening releasing its flaming red Qi forward and to the space between your shoulder blades to protect you.

☐ Breathe deeply while you imagine the continuous radiant, warm red light.

☐ Now turn your mind to the lung areas (the Metal Element) opening to the chest's front, back, and sides while a bright white light emerges, forming a shield around the body.

☐ Continue breathing deeply and slowly while seeing the lungs expanding their Qi, so it fills up the organs and overflows.

☐ We are now going to protect the right side of the body by expanding the liver's bright green light (the Wood Element). See the flow of this protective Qi layering around the right side of the body while continuing with deep abdomen breathing.

☐ Keep your eyes closed and visualize the colors coming together: yellow from the earth, red from the protective heart center, white from the lungs, blue from the kidneys, and green from the liver. These colors come together in a protective guarding layer around your body.

☐ Bring your mind back to your breathing and stay grounded for a few cycles of relaxed breaths with your hands on your belly.

☐ Now, return each color to its organ: Visualize the yellow to the spleen, the red to the heart, the white to the lungs, the blue to the kidneys, and the green to the liver.

☐ With your hands on the belly, massage your belly slowly in small circles. See the beautiful colors in and around the body protecting you.

Chapter 7:

How to Integrate Techniques for Reducing Anxiety into Daily Life

As you begin to realize that every different type of music, everybody's individual music, has its rhythm, life, language, and heritage, you realize how life changes, and you learn how to be more open and adaptive to what is around us. —Yo-Yo Ma

Qi in Everyday Life

Qi is energy, and we function on energy. What is your Qi rhythm? How could you harmonize your unique Qi with your busy schedule? In this chapter, I guide you to find your own Qi music in breathing, regular Qigong practices, and acupressure to revive the Qi music you were born with.

This chapter illustrates how to incorporate some of the techniques from earlier chapters, plus some new ones, into your daily life on the go.

Qi is energy, vibrating and present in our bodies. Let's briefly remind ourselves of the life force in our bodies.

Notice Your Energy

☐ Find somewhere quiet where you can be calm.

☐ Stand with feet shoulder-width apart.

- [ ] Breathe deeply in and out a couple of times.

- [ ] Rub your arm vigorously.

- [ ] Do you feel the friction and your arm heating up? It is electrical energy, your bio-electricity, your power.

Our body cells are atoms vibrating with energy, and by rubbing your arm, you have activated that energy. Let's do another short practice to wake up our Qi and move it to the belly.

Awaken Your Energy

- [ ] Rub your hands briskly until they are warm.

- [ ] Clap your hands vigorously to activate the nerves and get them to release more electrical energy.

- [ ] Hold your hands in front of you, not quite touching. Move your mind to the space between your hands. Do you feel the electrostatic friction between your hands? A buzzing, tingling, or warmth? It is your Qi.

- [ ] Keep breathing deeply and slowly.

- [ ] Hold your hands in front of your belly so that your palms face each other as if you're holding a ball. Tune in to the sensations in your palms. With practice, you may find that you feel warmth or tingling and a feeling of connection or magnetism between your palms.

- [ ] Slowly move your palms a tiny bit further away from each other, then a tiny bit closer. As you pulse the palms back and forth, you can sometimes feel the energy between them getting a little denser.

- [ ] While breathing deeply, bring your hands to your belly and gather the energy there. You might feel a little warmth or a sensation.

Quick Relief Exercises

You can use your breath and acupoints to help you release anxiety quickly.

Breath as Anxiety Relief Tool

Box breathing is our go-to technique, as we can do it anywhere in public or private. Refer to Chapter 3 for a detailed description. Here is a short reminder: Place your hand on your navel. Breathe in for four counts. Hold for four counts. Breathe out for four counts. Hold for four counts.

Peace breathing is another one-minute exercise that may help us calm down amid the most chaotic day. Do this on the train or bus, even during a difficult conversation. Take a few slow breaths, and with each inhale, in your mind, say to yourself: I am. With each exhale, say: at peace. Repeat as much as you can to help relieve tension.

Ten-to-zero breathing is a two-minute practice; we count down from ten to zero, doing a full breath (in and out) for each count. Inhale slowly, then relax as you extend the exhale to about the count of 10, or whatever is comfortable for you. Continue in this way until you reach zero and feel the relaxation in your body.

Body relaxation breathing does what the name says: We deliberately relax our bodies. Wherever we are, commuting, in a meeting, or having a quick lunch break, we can do body relaxation breathing. We are often unaware that we hold tension in a specific body part. Check your body for tension, then consciously relax the areas that need it. Relax the facial muscles. Wrinkle your forehead and relax. Move the brows as if questioning something and relax them. Squint your eyes and relax. Slack your jaw and open your mouth slightly.

Roll your shoulders and drop them away from your ears. Rest your arms on your lap, your hands open and fingers slightly parted. Uncross your ankles and relax into your chair. Let your knees open and feel how your legs and feet become heavier. Breathe deeply in and out through your nose.

Progressive muscle relaxation is a variation of the previous breathing technique. For this one, you need a little privacy. Lie down and take a few deep breaths. We start at the feet and work up the body to the face. Breathe in and tense the feet deliberately. Really work on contracting the muscles in the foot, toes, arch, and the angle of your foot. Breathe out while you relax all the muscles in the foot. Be aware of how the toes, arch, etc., relax as you slowly breathe out.

Repeat this with every body part: legs, knees, pelvic area, belly, chest, arms, hands, shoulder, neck, and all the different parts of the face. Contract the muscles intensely while you breathe in, and relax the muscles completely while you breathe out.

Lion's breath requires more privacy, so find a quiet moment and lock the door if possible. Sit comfortably and breathe in deeply through your nose. The idea is to fill the belly with air. Now, open your mouth as wide as possible and breathe with the sound HAAA. Repeat several times to help get rid of your tension.

Acupressure as Anxiety Relief Tool

Here are some acupressure points which can be used on the go. Remember to breathe slowly and deeply when massaging or pressing the point.

The **Hall of Impression** (*Yin Tang*) point (M-HN-3) is right between our eyebrows. You can do this privately, but, if necessary, you can apply pressure to this point even in a busy office while "studying" a document on your desk. Sit comfortably and if you can, close your eyes. Otherwise, soft-focus a few inches ahead of you, not seeing anything. Find the spot with your index finger or thumb and gently press this point for about 30 seconds. Move your finger in slow, small circles.

Heaven Gate point can also be pressed in public without attracting much attention. This point is in the upper shell, just under the curve of the ear. It might help to look in a mirror until you are familiar with the spot. The cartilage forms a triangle, and the spot is right at its tip in a small hollow. Apply firm pressure and move in small circles for a few minutes.

The **Heavenly Crevice**, *Tianliao* (TW-15), points are on top of your shoulder bone. When you're on the go or at your desk, this acupressure point is great to help relieve tension and anxiety. Curve your fingers over your shoulders like a hook. Use your fingertips to press the point on the top of your shoulder bone. Take three or four slow breaths, then release.

The **Great Rushing** (LIV-3) points are discussed in more detail in Chapter 4, but here is a quick reminder to do under your desk. It's on the top of your feet. Slip your shoe off; with your right heel, press, and massage into the LIV-3 point in the hollow where the big toe and the next toe intersect. Repeat with the other foot. The Great Rushing points are powerful and help with more than anxiety relief. Pressing these points may also help with pain and insomnia.

Inner Gate (P-6) is on the arm, and we refer to it in Chapter 6. This gate helps build protective energy internally. Stimulating the Inner Gate also helps with nausea and pain. Turn your hand, palm facing up. Find the point by placing three fingers from your free hand on the wrist crease. This point lies between the tendons. Press firmly into the spot and then massage in small circles.

Playful Qigong practices may help when anxiety grabs you on challenging days.

Tapping or knocking the chest is excellent for getting rid of too much heart energy, the pent-up Qi that feels heavy in the heart and makes you feel like you'll explode. Inhale, hold your breath for a second or two. Knock your fists up and down the sternum in the center of your chest. Continue tapping up and down the chest as you exhale through your mouth. It can be effective for releasing anxiety and emotional tension on the spot.

Let the balloon go with your eyes closed. Take deep breaths, holding an imaginary helium-type balloon. Breathe out your anxiety through your mouth into an imaginary balloon. Tie the balloon, hold it by a string, lift it high into the air and let it go. With your eyes closed, watch it go higher and higher and further away. Watch it become smaller and smaller; so small it's only a dot on the horizon.

Routines to Relieve Anxiety

The following practices combine the techniques discussed in this book: breathing, acupressure, and Qigong, and weave them into everyday life. They can make a meaningful contribution to our rushed and busy lives as we can do them anywhere and in limited spaces. Even a few minutes can go a long way in relieving anxiety. These techniques allow us to slow down our mind and body and build our energy reserves.

Getting Out of Bed

Picking Cherries

- Stand with your feet shoulder-width, knees bent, and tailbone tucked under.

- Reach your arms above your head. Stretch one up further, then the other, alternately looking up. Feel the gentle stretch at the base of the spine and in the muscles on either side of the spine.

- Slowly relax the arms down your sides. This stretch releases compression in the back and stretches through the ribs, opening the energy through the muscles involved in respiration.

- Repeat a few times.

After my shower, I do a few more exercises. They take only a minute or two but set me up for the day.

- Start rubbing your hands vigorously. Feel the heat building up as you stimulate the cells to release energy.

A facial massage stimulates blood flow and Qi, refreshes, and prepares me for a busy day.

☐ Place your palms on your closed eyes for about half a minute.

☐ Massage upward along your cheeks on either side of your nose to your eyebrows. There are acupressure points there, including one which some call Facial Beauty (St-3).

☐ Next, sweep the palm of your hand across your forehead.

☐ Tap lightly with your fingertips around the jaw.

☐ Brush your fingers through your hair over the scalp, from the forehead down to the back of the neck.

☐ Tap the back of the neck with your fingertips, or interlace your fingers and do thumb circles there. The points here are good for releasing stress and tension.

☐ Use alternate hands to squeeze your neck. Squeeze and release, squeeze and release.

☐ Massage your ears between your fingers and thumb. There are acupoints all over your ears, so it's like you're massaging your whole body.

☐ Shake your hands, removing the tension in your arms and fingers.

The spine is vital to maintaining a healthy posture and central nervous system; sometimes, the spine can be compressed during sleep. It is a good idea to energize the spine.

☐ Use one hand at a time and tap lightly around the top vertebrae rhythmically. Change hands and tap away.

☐ Then tap either side of the lower spine up and down the lower back and kidney area. Chinese medicine considers the kidneys to be like the batteries of the body. The lower back tapping boosts energy to help you get ready for the day.

☐ End your practice as you began: Stand comfortably but with the spine aligned and your hands beside your body.

☐ Breathe in deeply and out slowly.

☐ Finally, inhale and raise your arms to the top of your head.

☐ Exhale and slowly float your fingertips down the front line of your body without touching, drawing energy through your head, heart, and belly. Feel the vitality in your body and the positivity in your mind. You are ready to have a good day!

Headaches

Often, tension and anxiety may manifest as a headache. Here are a few acupoints and Qigong exercises to relieve headaches. It's always a good idea to drink plenty of fluids if you have a headache. When our bodies are dehydrated, the tissues lose moisture and contract. The brain also shrinks, and as it pulls away from the skull, the nerves become active and cause pain.

Persistent or regular headaches should be checked with your physician.

Try the following pressure point:

☐ Find *Large Intestine *(LI-4), on top of the hand, in the web valley where the bones of the thumb and the index finger meet. It is right at the bone points, not in the fleshy part of the web. Feel around it: It will usually feel tender when you're at the right spot.

☐ This point helps to regulate the face and head area.

☐ Press or circle massage the point with the thumb of the other hand for about a minute while breathing slowly and relaxed.

☐ Switch hands.

*This point is not recommended for pregnant women.

Chin Circles

Try a few chin circles for headaches and neck tension.

☐ Bring your hands together behind you, palms facing your back. Modify this position to feel comfortable. You can have the hands a bit up or down. If this position is uncomfortable, hold one arm or have the arms beside the body.

☐ Take the usual Qigong position: Feet shoulder-width apart and knees slightly bent. Consciously, relax your jaw.

☐ Bring your chin down to your chest, pressing palms together but shoulders relaxed.

☐ Bring your chin around to the front of your right shoulder and look down toward your right toes.

☐ Gently, do little tiny chin circles right in front of the shoulder. You should be able to feel it in the opposite shoulder and neck, like a deep-tissue massage.

☐ Breathe deeply in and out to release tension. Relax the shoulders and modify the movements to what feels right for you.

☐ Reverse the circle.

☐ Keep your chin down and move back to the front center.

☐ Now bring your chin in front of your left shoulder and look to your left toes.

☐ Repeat the slow movements, making small circles with your chin. Feel the release on the opposite shoulder and neck.

- Bring your hands down to the sides and feel the movement of energy through your neck and shoulders.

Minutes Before a Difficult Meeting

Do you also have that sinking feeling in the pit of your stomach before a difficult meeting? Or do you dread an unpleasant task? Find somewhere private ahead of the meeting; even the restroom will do. Just be quiet for a moment. Notice where your stress is: Is your heart racing, your jaw locked, or your neck tight? Do you feel a blinding headache coming? Just notice and slow your breathing.

- Stand with feet shoulder-width apart. Consciously, relax your mind.

- Breathe deeply in and out. If your chest is tight, hold one hand on your belly and the other on your chest. This simple stance may help you move your breath to your belly.

- Inhale slowly and deeply, moving the breath in three steps: into the belly, onto the ribs, and then the chest.

- Exhale slowly, first from the chest, then the ribs, and lastly, the belly.

- Do you still feel some tightness or shortness of breath despite breathing in steps? At the top of the inhale, just pause and wait for the exhale to happen all by itself. When the exhale starts, relax and melt into it. With each breath, relax deeper.

- Inhale deeply: belly, ribs, and chest.

- Exhale slowly: chest, ribs, and belly.

The following quick practice may help to balance your emotions in minutes. Steal a few moments before a stressful meeting and find somewhere to be still.

- Inhale and exhale deeply and slowly.

- Find the Sea of Tranquility, *Shanzhong* (CV-17), on the bone in the center of the chest. It is about three thumbs width up from the base of the bone.

- Press for about a minute while taking three or four relaxed breaths.

Alternatively, you can press the Inner Gate (P-6) for about a minute. Chapter 6 explains where to find this point on the inner arm, three fingers up from the wrist crease.

Insomnia

When your mind is busy, it is hard for the body to relax. Sometimes, consciously trying to sleep causes even more tension. Make sure you are comfortable in your bedroom with all devices switched off. Try the following techniques and see what works best for you.

There are pressure points all over your feet, and massaging them can help to draw energy down the body and away from your busy mind. A foot massage before bedtime can help you calm down.

- Sit comfortably and use your thumb to massage the whole of each foot by pressing and releasing. Massage along the arch of the foot, the ankles and toes, and in the webbing between the big and second toes.

- Next, press with your thumb up the inside leg and along the bone to three fingers above the ankle bone. This is the *Three Yin Intersection *(SP 6) and is often recommended for better sleep. Breathe slowly and relaxed.

This point is not recommended for pregnant women.

Wind Pool or *Fengchi* (GB-20) is another acupressure point that may help the body relax. It can help with headaches and improve sleep.

- [ ] Interlock the fingers and take your hands behind your neck.

- [ ] Put your thumbs at the bottom of your skull. There is a kind of archway where the head and the neck connect. Feel the little dip on either side.

- [ ] Press firmly, using small circular movements. You can also massage these points up and down.

- [ ] Breathe deeply and notice how your body feels.

Sound breathing can guide your body into relaxation and calmness. It can contribute to falling asleep. Chapter 5 gives more detailed information on sound breathing. Here is the healing sound Triple Warmer that helps to relax the body and can also help with sleep.

- [ ] Stand with feet shoulder-width apart.

- [ ] Inhale, float your hands above your head, palms over your head.

- [ ] While you exhale, bring your hands down in front of your body and palms facing as with Pulling Down the Heavens, described in Chapter 5. However, make the HEEE sound as you exhale.

- [ ] Feel a wave of relaxation through the body.

- [ ] Repeat for about a minute or so.

Part of Your Everyday Life (Almost)

We constantly neglect our inner needs as we dart from one thing to the other with barely time to think. We often don't make time for ourselves. At one point in my Qigong journey, I was trying so hard to master the techniques to get my energy flowing freely that I got stressed. Yes, I fell back into my negative default: Trying to be perfect and getting anxious!

This was when I discovered the value of a face-to-face class. My teacher noticed my stress and connected the dots. I was using my Qi to gain more Qi! Without any judgment, she guided me back to slow breathing. The penny eventually dropped: I did not have to achieve anything in Qigong. There are no exams, no level to reach. All I had to do was be with my mind, breath, and body, allowing the Qi to flow.

I have found that I need daily practice to stay breath-fit and stress-free. Daily breathing and energy work is my way to keep my body and mind ready to handle those unforeseen crises that unavoidably cross one's path from time to time.

What can be better than having a few private moments early in the morning in bed, listening to the passing traffic, and doing box breathing? My morning belly breathing has become my anchor for the day.

On challenging days, I do acupressure in preparation for upcoming stressful events. It takes less than five minutes but helps for much longer. It has been a lifesaver many times.

Additionally, I do online Qigong practices before bedtime to relax and sleep better. There are many five to ten minutes videos available, and it might help to try out a few until you find an online space that suits your needs. I developed my own bedtime practices and will share them with you later.

Keep notes at the end of the day. Jot down what worked for you that day. I hope you find your way to calmness right there in your high-speed life.

Some Final Thoughts

This book focuses on anxiety relief techniques rather than anxiety and its causes. I'd like it to help people as much as possible. Please submit a review where you purchased it, which will help people to know about it. Thank you.

You will find many books on anxiety and its psychological impact. This book has a different angle. It guides you to find relief inside yourself, in your breath, and in your mind, regardless of the cause of your anxiety.

The problem is that most of us tend to ignore simple solutions, especially if they come free. We tend to believe in the more complex answers to life's questions. Confucius said, "Life is really simple, but we insist on making it complicated." It is human to expect complex solutions, but this book, based on traditional Chinese medicine, does the opposite. It aims to describe healing practices straightforwardly and explain how they work.

By breathing deeply and consciously, your body's parasympathetic nervous system kicks in, and the body relaxes. When the body is relaxed, it signals to the brain that danger has passed. The brain reacts by releasing endorphins, the feel-good hormones that lessen anxiety.

Acupressure should not be confused with acupuncture, although it uses the same acupoints. Acupressure does not use needles; you can do acupressure on yourself to increase blood flow, bring fresh oxygen, and allow free energy flow in your body.

It is not a substitute for medical care but a complementary approach to staying healthy. Western medicine increasingly supports acupressure and breathing techniques as treatments alongside medical treatment. They are beneficial in preventative health practices and addressing many chronic health issues.

Pressing acupoints may also help to unblock congested emotions: those feelings, pain, or anger we sometimes harbor in our bodies for many years.

This book offers a practical guide to the most powerful pressure points and breathing techniques to address anxiety. The author knows the challenges of the 21st century: career, family, and relationships. He compiled a list of quick techniques, especially for a busy individual, and is grateful to Caroline at LessStressMoreEnergy.com for the wonderful Qigong classes and the inspiration for many on-the-go techniques.

The beauty is that you can do these breathing techniques and press the appropriate anxiety relief points sitting behind your desk or on the bus without attracting attention. They are truly designed for an on-the-go lifestyle.

Anxiety usually builds up over a long time, and often it has been cemented into our psyches before we see it and seek help. These quick techniques may help at the moment and give immediate relief, but only by continuing with relaxing practices can we begin to address deep-rooted and long-term anxiety.

Qigong can go a long way in helping you to become calmer. Qigong is a traditional Eastern art that coordinates body-posture, movement, breathing, and meditation to improve physical and emotional health. It is gentle and allows you to slowly build the relaxing techniques into your muscle and mind memory. With repetition, they become second nature—your natural default to handle life's crises. Qigong's meditative movements calm the mind and automatically build up the energy reserves necessary for our busy days.

Inherent to breathing, acupressure and Qigong is Qi, the body's life force that keeps us going, along with nutrients, oxygen, and fluids. Qi is not an alien concept; it is an analog to electrical currents, microwaves, heart, muscle, and brain waves expressed as ECG, EMG, and EEG.

Qi is the energy in our bodies. Our body cells are atoms vibrating with energy, and through the simple practices in this book, you can learn to activate the energy, open the pathways through which it flows, and help to combat anxiety.

It might astonish you that we can spread our Qi, positive or negative, to people around us. We all know someone whose company drains us, leaving us exhausted and anxious. We can shield ourselves from negative energy, and this book tells you how to begin to lift your own anxiety and protect yourself energetically and cultivate an intention to protect positive energy.

What's more, you can learn to project your positive Qi to the world and be a happier human being. I wish you greater lightness and happiness in your life to come.

References

Acupuncture Points. (2017, October 3). *How to locate the Heart 8 Shaofu (Lesser Palace)* [Video]. YouTube. https://www.youtube.com/watch?v=XrT9CRs7Dpg

Benisek, A. (n.d.), *What to know about mouth breathing.* WebMD. https://www.webmd.com/oral-health/mouth-breathing

Berry, W. (2019, July 21). *You aren't built to be happy.* Psychology Today. https://www.psychologytoday.com/us/blog/the-second-noble-truth/201907/you-arent-built-be-happy

Brennan, D. (n.d.). *What is box breathing?* WebMD. https://www.webmd.com/balance/what-is-box-breathing

Bullock, B. G., (2019, October 31). *What focusing on the breath does to your brain.* Greater Good Magazine. https://greatergood.berkeley.edu/article/item/what_focusing_on_the_breath_does_to_your_brain

Burgess, L. (2018, November 23). *Foot massage techniques and benefits.* Medical News Today. https://www.medicalnewstoday.com/articles/323790

Caroline Allen. (2022, May 7). *Headache & neck tension release* [Video]. YouTube https://www.youtube.com/watch?v=f8ePRN4hFmo

Campbell, A. (2018). *NLP Made Easy: How to use neuro-linguistic programming to change your life.* Hay House, Inc.

Chen, K. (2019). *Acupuncture point Shenmen "Spirit Gate."* Tai Chi Acupuncture & Wellness Center. https://www.taichi-wellness.com/events_articles/events_articles_cont.php?id=298&subject=Acupuncture+Point+Shenmen+%22Spirit+Gate

Chopra. (2018, August 28). *Top 30 Deepak Chopra Quotes.* https://chopra.com/articles/top-30-deepak-chopra-quotes

Chung, Y., Chen, J., Ko, K. (2016). Spleen function and anxiety in Chinese Medicine: A Western perspective. *Chinese Medicine* Volume 7, 110-123. https://doi.org/10.4236/cm.2016.73012

Cirino, E. (n.d.). *8 Pressure points on your hands.* Healthline. https://www.healthline.com/health/hand-pressure-points

Cohen, M. R. (n.d.). *8 Powerful ancient Qigong exercises for cultivating healing energy in the body.* Conscious Lifestyle. https://www.consciouslifestylemag.com/qigong-exercises-healing-energy/

Curran, J. (2008, April 5). The Yellow Emporer's Classic of Internal Medicine. *The British Medical Journal.* https://doi.org/10.1136/bmj.39527.472303.4E

Daling acupoint: PC7 acupuncture point Or pericardium 7 (P7). (2021, March 8). Peak Massager. https://www.peakmassager.com/pc-7-acupuncture-point/

Deadman, P., Al-Khafaji, M., Baker, K. (1998). *A manual of acupuncture.* The Journal of Chinese Medicine Publications

Directing energy with Qigong. (2020, May 24). Long White Cloud Qigong. https://www.longwhitecloudqigong.com/directing-energy-with-qigong/

Earth, late summer, spleen and stomach. (n.d.). Traditional Acupuncture Clinic. https://www.tcmacupuncturelex.com/earth-late-summer-spleen-and-stomach/

18 Benefits of deep breathing and how to breathe deeply? (2015). OnePowefulWord. https://www.onepowerfulword.com/2010/10/18-benefits-of-deep-breathing-and-how.html

Estrada, J. (2018, November 23). *How to use Qigong meditation to harness the healing energy of your body.* Well+Good.

https://www.wellandgood.com/qigong-meditation/#main-content

Fletcher, J. (2020, December 21). *The 10 best pressure points for the ears.* Medical   News   Today. https://www.medicalnewstoday.com/articles/ear-pressure-points

Fowler, P. (n.d.). *Breathing techniques for stress relief.* WebMD. https://www.webmd.com/balance/stress-management/stress-relief-breathing-techniques

Francesco Garri Garripoli. (2016, July 23*). Qigong documentary overview by Francesco   Garri   Garripoli*   [Video].   YouTube https://www.youtube.com/watch?v=Y7y_BMYaCGM

Gumenick, N. (2004, March 5). *Using the spirits of the points: The heart meridian.*   Acupuncture   Today. https://www.acupuncturetoday.com/mpacms/at/article.php?id=28406

Hanh, T. N [@thichnhathanh] (2018, April 6). *Breath is the bridge that connects life to consciousness, the bridge that unites your body to your thoughts. Whenever your mind becomes scattered, use your breath as the means to take hold of your mind again* [Tweet]. Twitter. https://twitter.com/thichnhathanh/status/982234163703984129

Healthline Editorial Team. (n.d.). *How to massage your pressure points.* https://www.healthline.com/health/pain-relief/how-to-massage-your-pressure-points

Holden, L (2022, February 9). *6 Ways to improve your sleep using Qigong principles.* Holden Qigong. https://www.holdenqigong.com/6-ways-to-improve-your-sleep-using-qi-gong-principles

Holden, L. (2020, July). *Qigong: 30-day challenge with Lee Holden. 30 short workouts.* Udemy. https://www.udemy.com/course/qi-gong-30-day-challenge-with-lee-holden-30-short-workouts

Holden QiGong. (2022, March 17). *8-Minute headache relief routine* [Video]. YouTube. https://www.youtube.com/watch?v=g8kvb8zCW7E

Holden QiGong. (2021, April 22). *How to remove negative energy and clear energy blocks.* Holden Qigong [Video]. You Tube. https://www.youtube.com/watch?v=R-QAydg7QAs

Holden QiGong. (2020, November 12). *3 Simple Qigong exercises for fast and natural stress relief* [Video]. YouTube. https://www.youtube.com/watch?v=M_uN05H12PE

Hoshaw, C. (2021, February 25). *Body awareness: How to deepen your connection with your body.* Healthline. https://www.healthline.com/health/mind-body/body-awareness

Iftikar, N. (2019, July 30). *7 Pressure points for nausea.* Healthline. https://www.healthline.com/health/pressure-points-for-nausea

Janice Tucker. (2020, July 30). *Qigong for protection from negative people or surroundings / Qigong for beginners.* Space to Relax. [Video]. You Tube. https://www.youtube.com/watch?v=ONYWi8Iw8wM

Kauffmann, J. (2020, February 18). *Mobilizing clarity and purpose with Kidney 1.* Mend. https://mendacupuncture.com/mobilizing-clarity-and-purpose-with-kidney-1/

Kinder, W. (n.d.). *Waves of breath.* MindfullyADD. https://mindfullyadd.com/waves-of-breath/

Kirkwood, J. (2015, November 18). *Master of the seas.* Five Element Acupressure. https://www.acupressure.com.au/wprss/?tag=grandfather-grandson

Kruse, J., Lee, S. (n.d.), *Biopotential electrode sensors in ECG/EEG/EMG systems.* Analog Devices. https://www.analog.com/en/technical-articles/biopotential-electrode-sensors-ecg-eeg-emg.html

Kseny. (2018, August 10). *5 Minute Qigong routine to wake you up. Qigong with Kseny* [Video]. YouTube. https://www.youtube.com/watch?v=dzsWJzep86c

Lipton B. (2005). *The biology of belief: Unleashing the power of consciousness, matter and miracles.* Mountain of Love

Liu B. (2017). Integrative Views of the Heart in Chinese and Western Medicine. *Integr Med Int*, (4), 46-51. https://doi.org/10.1159/000466695

Liu, Z. W., Shu, J., Tu, J. Y., Zhang, C. H, Hong, J. (2017). Liver in the Chinese and Western Medicine. *Integr Med Int*, (4), 39-45. https://doi.org/10.1159/000466694

Long White Cloud Qigong. (2019, March 24). *Feeling electrical energy in your body in your Qigong exercise* [Video]. YouTube. https://www.youtube.com/watch?v=MD3YOYkndh4

Lorenz, R. (2014). Health Benefits of Singing: A Perspective from Traditional Chinese Medicine and Chi Kung. *The Phenomenon Of Singing*, (9), 154-166. https://journals.library.mun.ca/ojs/index.php/singing/article/view/1030/884

Macrobiotics Today. (2021, December 17). *Acupressure point Kidney 1* [Video] YouTube. https://www.youtube.com/watch?v=tGrLpH5yhew

Mini-relaxation exercises: A quick fix in stressful moments. (2012, November 10). Harvard Health Publishing. https://www.health.harvard.edu/healthbeat/mini-relaxation-exercises-a-quick-fix-in-stressful-moments

Nick Loffree Bioenergetic Health. (2018, July 3). *Protect your energy—Qigong exercises for psychic protection—empath training* [Video]. YouTube. https://www.youtube.com/watch?v=pOuQbNE9r00

Neill, M. (2013), *Supercoach: 10 Secrets to transform anyone's life.* Hay House UK

Newman, K. M. (2020, November 10). *Is the way you breathe making you anxious?* Greater Good Magazine. https://greatergood.berkeley.edu/article/item/is_the_way_you _breathe_making_you_anxious

Nwanegbo-Ben, J. (2016). Quantum physics and ESP (An Epistemic Resolution). *International Journal of Philosophy.* 4(3), 11-17. doi:10.11648/j.ijp.20160403.11

Pericardium 7 (n.d.). Ageless Herbs. https://agelessherbs.com/pericardium-7

Puddicombe, A. (2016, September 27). *The Headspace guide to meditation and mindfulness: How mindfulness can change your life in ten minutes a day.* St Martin's Griffen New York

Qi & Prana with Haunani. (2017, September 11). *Spleen 3 & 4 acupressure point finder* [Video] YouTube. https://www.youtube.com/watch?v=X1NIE5I1UYI

Qigong Less Stress More Energy. (n.d.). *Home* [Facebook page]. Facebook. https://www.facebook.com/lessstressmoreenergy/?_rdc=2&_ rdr

Qigong Meditation. (2022, June 13). *Healing headache / Qigong massage movements daily routine / 5 minus* [Video]. YouTube. https://www.youtube.com/watch?v=RyrQ-pYIXW0

Raypole, C. (n.d.). *6 Pressure points for anxiety relief.* Healthline. https://www.healthline.com/health/pressure-points-for-anxiety

Reed Gach, M. (1990, November 1). *Acupressure potent points and acupressure for emotional healing.* Bantam Books.

Reid, T. (n.d.). *The internal organs in Traditional Chinese Medicine.* Sun Herbal. https://sunherbal.com/basic-page/internal-organs-traditional-chinese-medicine

Reninger, E. (2019, January 26). *Lao gong Pericardium 8*. Learn Religions. https://www.learnreligions.com/acupressure-treasures-lao-gong-pericardium-8-3182279

Scaccia, A. (2018, January 8). *The acupressure points for inducing labour.* Healthline. https://www.healthline.com/health/pregnancy/acupressure-points-inducing-labor

Seaver, M. (2021, June 23). *Email apnea is a real thing—Here's how to stop holding your breath while you work (and feel less stressed).* Real Simple. https://www.realsimple.com/health/preventative-health/email-apnea-holding-breath-while-working

Sengar, C. (2020, May 4). *Foot massage for insomnia: Get over sleeplessness by massaging your feet before bed.* Onlymyhealth. https://www.onlymyhealth.com/foot-massage-to-get-sleep-at-night-1588586596

Shaofu Acupoint: HT8 Acupuncture point or Heart 8. (2021, March 7). Peak Massager. https://www.peakmassager.com/ht-8-acupuncture-point/

Siffet, S. (2018, December 27). *Can TCM help anxiety and depression?* One Medical. https://www.onemedical.com/blog/get-well/tcm-anxiety-depression/

Spiegelman, M. (n.d.-a). *How to stop other people's negativity like a sponge (Part 1).* Beacons of Change. https://www.beaconsofchange.com/stop-absorbing-negativity/

Spiegelman, M. (n.d.-b). *How to stop other people's negativity like a sponge (Part 2).* Beacons of Change. https://www.beaconsofchange.com/stop-absorbing-negativity-2/

Steber, C. (2017, December 26). *11 Subtle signs someone may be uncomfortable around you.* Bustle. https://www.bustle.com/p/11-

subtle-signs-someone-may-be-uncomfortable-around-you-7662695

The benefits of slow breathing and why it's vital to health. (2017, October 30). Moonbird. https://www.moonbird.life/magazine/slow-breathing-for-health/

The fire element. (n.d.). Thomson Chinese Medicine. https://www.thomsontcm.sg/articles/the-fire-element-in-tcm/

The origins of western and eastern medicine. (2019, February 20). Medibank. https://www.medibank.com.au/livebetter/health-brief/health-insights/the-origins-of-western-and-eastern-medicine/

Traveling the energetic highway: What are meridians? (2022). Center Point Healing. https://www.centerpointhealing.com/hyattsville/traveling-the-energetic-highway-what-are-meridians/

Vanbuskirk, S. (n.d.). *How emotions and organs are connected in traditional Chinese medicine.* Verywell Mind. https://www.verywellmind.com/emotions-in-traditional-chinese-medicine-88196

Walker, T. (2021, October 12). *How to boost—or chill—your energy with your breath.* Shine. https://advice.theshineapp.com/articles/how-to-boost-or-chill-your-energy-with-your-breath/

Yoqi Yoga and Qigong. (2017, June 1). *Daily Qigong routine* [Video]. YouTube. https://www.youtube.com/watch?v=nmmNWj9YtAw

Yuen, C. (n.d.). *How to fall asleep in 10, 60, or 120 seconds.* Healthline. https://www.healthline.com/health/healthy-sleep/fall-asleep-fast

Zadok, F. (2021, March 5). *Qigong—The basics of breath.* Aquatic Exercise Association. https://aeawave.org/Articles-More/Better-Health/ArtMID/1614/ArticleID/164/QiGong-The-Basics-of-Breath

Printed in Great Britain
by Amazon

16454341R00068